# Advanced Pediatric Craniocervical Surgery

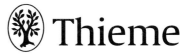

# Advanced Pediatric Craniocervical Surgery

Douglas L. Brockmeyer, M.D.
Professor
Division of Pediatric Neurosurgery
Department of Neurosurgery
University of Utah
Primary Children's Medical Center
Salt Lake City, Utah

Thieme
New York • Stuttgart

Thieme Medical Publishers, Inc.
333 Seventh Ave.
New York, NY 10001

Editor: Tim Hiscock
Associate Editor: Birgitta Brandenburg
Consulting Editor: Esther Gumpert
Vice-President, Production and Electronic Publishing: Anne T. Vinnicombe
Editorial Assistant: Christine Freeman
Associate Marketing Director: Verena Diem
Sales Director: Ross Lumpkin
Chief Financial Officer: Peter van Woerden
President: Brian D. Scanlan
Compositor: Thomson Digital Services
Printer: Maple-Vail Book Manufacturing Group
Library of Congress Cataloging-in-Publication Data

Library of Congress Cataloging-in-Publication Data

Brockmeyer, Douglas L.
     Advanced pediatric craniocervical surgery / Douglas L. Brockmeyer.
          p. ; cm.
     Includes bibliographical references.
     ISBN 1-58890-396-6 (TMP : alk. paper) -- ISBN 3-13-132081-8 (GTV : alk. paper) 1.
Spine--Surgery. 2. Cervical vertebrae--Surgery. 3. Skull--Surgery. 4. Pediatric
orthopedics.
     [DNLM: 1. Spinal Diseases--surgery--Adolescent. 2. Spinal Diseases--surgery--Child. 3.
Spinal Diseases--surgery--Infant. 4. Cervical Vertebrae--abnormalities--Adolescent. 5.
Cervical Vertebrae--abnormalities--Child. 6. Cervical Vertebrae--abnormalities--Infant.
7. Cervical Vertebrae--surgery--Adolescent. 8. Cervical Vertebrae--surgery--Child. 9.
Cervical Vertebrae--surgery--Infant. 10. Occipital Bone--abnormalities--Adolescent. 11.
Occipital Bone--abnormalities--Child. 12. Occipital Bone--abnormalities--Infant. 13.
Occipital Bone--surgery--Adolescent. 14. Occipital Bone--surgery--Child. 15. Occipital
Bone--surgery--Infant. WE 725 B864a 2006] I. Title.
     RD768.B665 2006
     617.5'083--dc22
                                        2005021936

**Important note:** Medical knowledge is ever-changing. As new research and clinical experience broaden our
knowledge, changes in treatment and drug therapy may be required. The authors and editors of the material
herein have consulted sources believed to be reliable in their efforts to provide information that is complete
and in accord with the standards accepted at the time of publication. However, in the view of the possibility of
human error by the authors, editors, or publisher, of the work herein, or changes in medical knowledge, neither
the authors, editors, or publisher, nor any other party who has been involved in the preparation of this work,
warrants that the information contained herein is in every respect accurate or complete, and they are not
responsible for any errors or omissions or for the results obtained from use of such information. Readers are
encouraged to confirm the information contained herein with other sources. For example, readers are advised
to check the product information sheet included in the package of each drug they plan to administer to be
certain that the information contained in this publication is accurate and that changes have not been made in
the recommended dose or in the contraindications for administration. This recommendation is of particular
importance in connection with new or infrequently used drugs.
Some of the product names, patents, and registered designs referred to in this book are in fact registered
trademarks or proprietary names even though specific reference to this fact is not always made in the text.
Therefore, the appearance of a name without designation as proprietary is not to be construed as a
representation by the publisher that it is in the public domain.

Printed in the United States of America

5 4 3 2 1

TMP ISBN 1-58890-396-6
GTV ISBN 3 13 132081 8

This book is dedicated to my wife Debra Lynn, my chilren Meghan and Russell, and the children that I have had the privilege to serve in my capacity as a pediatric neurosurgeon.

*Douglas L. Brockmeyer, M.D.*

# Contents

## 2. Clinical Biomechanics of the Pediatric Craniocervical Junction and Subaxial Spine ........................27

Marcus L. Ware, Nalin Gupta, Peter P. Sun, and Douglas
L. Brockmeyer

## 3. Common Pathological Conditions of the Pediatric Craniovertebral Junction and Cervical Spine .........43

Douglas L. Brockmeyer

# Preface

When I began my career in Pediatric Neurosurgery, little or no emphasis was placed on the management of craniocervical disorders in children. Pediatric craniovertebral surgery seemed like no-man's land, an orphan subspecialty tucked between the arena of adult spine surgery and the shunt-dominated world of pediatric neurosurgery. Luckily, I had enjoyed extensive cervical spine experience during my residency and looked forward to the challenge of treating children with spinal disorders. Little did I know how unprepared I was. Each case that presented itself seemed more difficult than the last, and over the years I sought help from a variety of sources. Slowly but surely, I was able to determine what worked and what didn't, while managing an astounding array of challenging cases. Some techniques I used were borrowed from adult spine surgery, some were planned specifically for pediatric use, and others were made up on the spot. The sum of those experiences and techniques are contained within this volume.

I have asked several other experts in pediatric spine surgery to discuss specific areas that are important in managing children with craniocervical disorders. The result, I hope, is a volume where the principles and techniques for managing pediatric craniocervical problems are covered in a single source. My intent here is not to be dogmatic but to share my experience and to encourage readers toward developing solutions on their own. Ultimately, I hope pediatric spine surgery will shed its orphan status and the techniques discussed in this book will be applied to the considerable challenges these patients represent.

## Acknowledgments

I gratefully acknowledge my surgical mentor, Dr. Ronald Apfelbaum, a wonderful teacher and innovator, who taught me that no problem is unsolvable. Also, I thank my partners, Dr. Marion Walker and Dr. John Kestle, for their help and encouragement over the years, as well as the other members of the Department of Neurosurgery, including our chairman, Dr. William Couldwell.

I wish to thank Kristin Kraus for her considerable help in editing and finalizing the manuscript, and Barbara Stephan for her wonderful illustrations.

*Douglas L. Brockmeyer, M.D.*

# Contributors

Kurtis Auguste, M.D.
Resident
Department of Neurological Surgery
University of California San Francisco Medical Center
San Francisco, California


Douglas L. Brockmeyer, M.D.
Professor
Division of Pediatric Neurosurgery
Department of Neurosurgery
University of Utah
Primary Children's Medical Center
Salt Lake City, Utah


Mark S. Dias, M.D., F.A.A.P.
Associate Professor of Neurosurgery
Vice Chair of Clinical Neurosurgery
Chief of Pediatric Neurosurgery
Milton S. Hershey Medical Center
Hershey, Pennsylvania


Nalin Gupta, M.D., Ph.D.
Assistant Professor of Neurological Surgery
   and Dennis Bruce Dettmer Endowed Chair in Pediatric Neurosurgery
Department of Neurological Surgery
University of California San Francisco Medical Center
San Francisco, California

Peter P. Sun, M.D.
Director
Division of Neurosurgery
Children's Hospital Oakland
Oakland, California


Marcus L. Ware, M.D., Ph.D.
Resident
Department of Neurological Surgery
University of California San Francisco Medical Center
San Francisco, California

# 1

# Anatomy, Embryology, and Normal and Abnormal Development of the Craniovertebral Junction and Cervical Spine

**Mark S. Dias and Douglas L. Brockmeyer**

The craniovertebral junction (CVJ) and cervical spine are among the most complex areas of the spine, both anatomically and embryologically. Because these regions develop from several different embryonic components, the opportunities for anatomical variants and embryological malformations in this region abound. A working knowledge of the anatomy, embryology, and many abnormal variants involving the CVJ and cervical spine is crucial to properly identifying the congenital nature of these abnormalities and differentiating them from traumatic lesions, as well as navigating the surgical approaches to this region. This chapter reviews the normal anatomy of the bony and ligamentous structures of the CVJ and cervical spine, the normal developmental sequence that results in these complex structures, and the embryopathological substrate upon which the various developmental malformations in this region can be organized.

The chapter presents topics regarding the subaxial cervical spine before topics regarding the CVJ. Convention usually dictates that the more cranial anatomical elements are presented first. As the reader will become aware, however, the embryological theories regarding CVJ development are built upon the theories of subaxial cervical spine development, and therefore, the lower cervical anatomical elements are presented first in the interest of clarity.

## ◆ Anatomy of the Subaxial Cervical Spine

### Bony, Disk, and Ligamentous Anatomy

The third to sixth cervical vertebrae are regarded as typical vertebrae, and the seventh cervical vertebra is a transitional vertebra. Each of the vertebrae from C3 to C6 has a small, broad body and a large, triangular vertebral foramen. The spinous processes are short, are usually bifid, and may be palpable. At the junctions of the pedicles and lamina, each vertebra has a pillar that gives rise to the superior and inferior articular processes. These processes present horizontally oriented facets. The superior facets are directed upward and backward, and the inferior facets are directed downward and forward. From C3 to C6, each transverse process is pierced by a foramen transversarium. Small projections, or tubercles, emanate from the transverse processes.

The seventh cervical vertebra is a transitional vertebra because its long spinous process does not bifurcate but ends in a tubercle that gives attachment to the ligamentum nuchae. Its transverse process is large, and the foramen transversarium is small or even absent. Rarely, the vertebral artery passes through the foramen transversarium of C7. The costal process of C7 may develop separately and form a cervical rib.

The intervertebral disks are comprised of a central nucleus pulposus surrounded by the anulus fibrosus. The firm attachment of the intervertebral disks to the vertebral bodies constitutes a major supportive structure of the cervical spinal canal.

There are two main ligamentous attachments of the subaxial cervical spine. The anterior longitudinal ligament (ALL) runs along the anterior portion of the vertebral bodies and intervertebral disks, and the posterior longitudinal ligament (PLL) runs along the posterior portion of the same structures. They also are major supportive structures of the cervical spinal column. The superior extent of the ALL fuses to the anterior portion of the atlas, and the superior extent of the PLL fuses with the tectorial membrane. The ALL and the PLL both extend inferiorly to the sacrum.

The interspinous ligament, located between each spinous process from C3 to C7, is a minor supportive structure of the spinal column. The capsular ligaments surrounding the facet joints are also minor supportive structures.

### Vascular and Lymphatic Anatomy

The most important vascular structure in the subaxial cervical spine is the vertebral artery. The vertebral artery courses through the soft tissues of the neck until it pierces the foramen transversarium at C6 and extends to the foramen transversarium of C3. The paraspinous tissue and vertebral column are fed by small vertebral artery branches.

The lymphatic drainage of the subaxial cervical spine is primarily into retropharyngeal lymph nodes and the cervical lymphatic chain.

## ◆ Anatomy of the Craniovertebral Junction

### Bony and Ligamentous Anatomy

The bony portion of the CVJ is composed of the occipital bone, the atlas (C1), and the axis (C2) (**Fig. 1–1**, bony relationships). The occipital bone makes up the posterior membranous cranium as well as the inferior skull base. The fora-

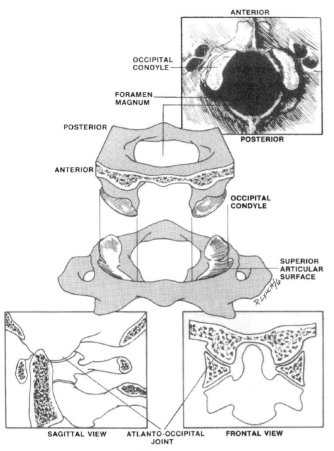

**Figure 1–1**    Anatomy of the craniocervical junction.

men magnum is formed from a ring of bony structures derived from the occipital bone and includes the inferior clivus anteriorly, the occipital condyles laterally, and the opisthion posteriorly. The paired hypoglossal canals originate in the anterolateral portion of the clivus superior to the occipital condyles. The paired occipital condyles articulate with the superior surface of the atlas facets, forming the atlanto-occipital facet joint.

The atlas consists of a bony ring that interfaces between the occipital condyles superiorly and the axis inferiorly. The atlas lacks a vertebral body and instead has arches that project anteriorly and posteriorly from the paired atlanto-occipital facet joints. The atlas articulates superiorly with the occiput and inferiorly with the axis; the inferior articular facets project medially and posteriorly to articulate with the superior facets of the axis. The atlas thus serves as a "washer" between the occipital condyles above and the axis below. The atlas has small tubercles bilaterally along the inner surface of the anterior arch for the attachment of the transverse ligament. The anterolateral portion of the atlas contains atretic transverse processes that house the vertebral foramina. A groove within the superior surface of the posterior arch of the atlas is present for the vertebral artery.

The axis is unique among the vertebrae in both its structure and its relationships with neighboring vertebrae. It is the only vertebra that has a bony projection from the vertebral body, namely, the odontoid process. The odontoid process articulates with the atlas superiorly; this articulation is lined with a circumferential synovial bursa. The axis articulates superiorly with the atlas via a horizontally oriented superior articular surface. The atlantoaxial joint is unique in the spine because it lacks an intervertebral disk; the C1–C2 interspace actually resembles a facet joint. Inferiorly, the axis articulates with the superior facet of C3.

The tectorial membrane, an important stabilizing structure of the atlanto-occipital joint, inserts into the anterior–inferior clivus and continues inferiorly as the PLL [**Fig. 1–2,** midsagittal magnetic resonance imaging (MRI)]. Other ligaments include the atlanto-occipital membrane, located in the dorsal aspect of the spinal canal, and the atlanto-occipital joint capsule supports. The atlantoaxial joint capsule articulations are lax and are reinforced laterally by the atlanto-occipital ligaments. The transverse ligament works as a check ligament to keep the odontoid snugly in place against the anterior arch of the atlas. Other minor ligaments that provide attachment of the axis to the occiput include the alar, apical dens, and cruciform ligaments.

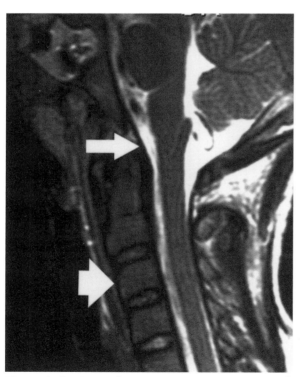

**Figure 1–2**    Sagittal magnetic resonance imaging showing the posterior longitudinal ligament (arrow) and the anterior longitudinal ligament (arrowhead).

## Vascular and Lymphatic Anatomy

The vascular supply of the CVJ comes from branches directly off the vertebral artery and from occipital branches of the carotid artery. A vascular arcade is formed around the odontoid process, but the embryological origin of the arcade precludes vascular communication between the base of the dens and the body of the axis. This anatomical relationship helps explain the origin of os odontoideum (OO) and the frequent nonunion of type II odontoid fractures.

The lymphatic drainage of the CVJ is primarily into retropharyngeal lymph nodes and the deep upper cervical lymphatic chain. The venous plexus around the odontoid drains into the suboccipital epidural sinuses and appears to have a direct communication with the pharyngovertebral veins. Pharyngovertebral–lymphovenous anastomoses have been described.[1] These communications are important in the genesis of Grisel's syndrome, an inflammatory or infectious retropharyngeal condition causing atlantoaxial rotatory subluxation.

## ◆ Embryology of the Cervical Spine

The normal development of the vertebral column includes six separate but overlapping phases: (1) gastrulation and the formation of the somitic mesoderm and notochord; (2) condensation of the somitic mesoderm to form the somites; (3) reorganization of the somites to form dermomyotome and sclerotome; (4) the membranous phase of somitic development and resegmentation of the somites to form the definitive vertebrae; (5) vertebral chondrification; and (6) vertebral ossification.

### Gastrulation and Formation of Somites and Notochord

During the first 2 weeks following fertilization, the human embryo undergoes several cell divisions and cellular rearrangements that ultimately form a blastocyst, a two-layered embryo suspended between the amnionic and yolk sacs (**Fig. 1–3**). Cells on the dorsal surface of the embryo adjacent to the amnionic cavity form the epiblast, whereas cells on the ventral surface adjacent to the yolk sac form the hypoblast.[2] By the end of the second week, the embryo thickens cranially to form the prochordal plate, the first morphological feature of craniocaudal orientation.

During the second week, the embryo undergoes gastrulation, which converts the embryo from a two- to a three-layered structure containing ectoderm, mesoderm, and endoderm. During early gastrulation, the primitive streak develops at the caudal end of the embryo and elongates cranially over 3 days (**Fig. 1–4**). At its full length, the primitive streak occupies the midline in the caudal half of the embryo. Subsequently the primitive streak becomes progressively shorter, regressing back toward the caudal pole of the embryo.[2] Throughout gastrulation cells of the epiblast migrate toward the primitive streak and invaginate through the primitive groove running the length of the primitive streak (**Fig. 1–4**). The first cells to ingress—while the primitive streak is still

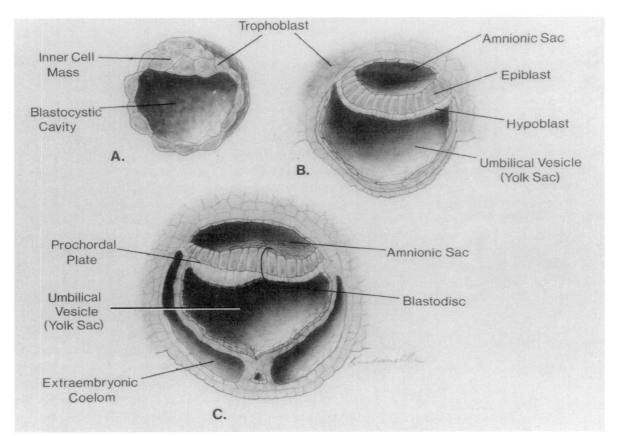

**Figure 1–3** Development of the blastocyst; midsagittal illustrations. **(A)** Continued proliferation of cells produces a sphere containing a blastocystic cavity surrounded by an eccentrically located inner cell mass and a surrounding ring of trophoblast cells. **(B)** The inner cell mass develops further into a two-layered structure, the blastodisk, containing the epiblast adjacent to the amnionic cavity and the hypoblast adjacent to the yolk sac. **(C)** With further development, the blastodisk thickens cranially to form the prochordal plate. (Reprinted with permission from Dias MS, Walker ML. The embryogenesis of complex dysraphic malformations: a disorder of gastrulation? Pediatr Neurosurg 1992;18:229–253.)

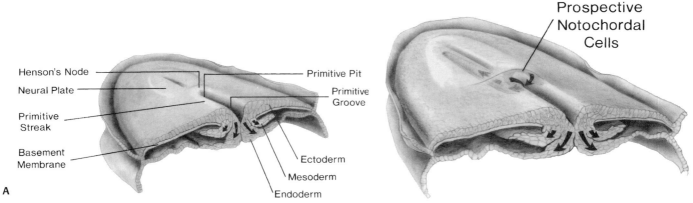

**Figure 1–4** Normal human gastrulation. **(A)** Prospective endodermal and mesodermal cells of the epiblast migrate toward the primitive streak and ingress (arrows) through the primitive groove to become the definitive endoderm and mesoderm. **(B)** Prospective notochordal cells in the cranial margin of Hensen's node will ingress through the primitive pit during primitive streak regression to become the notochordal process. (Reprinted with permission from Dias MS, Walker ML. The embryogenesis of complex dysraphic malformations: a disorder of gastrulation? Pediatr Neurosurg 1992;18:229–253.)

elongating—give rise to the embryonic endoderm.[3–5] Later, as the streak begins to regress toward the caudal pole, endodermal cells are replaced by prospective mesodermal cells that insinuate themselves between the epiblast and the newly formed endoderm. These ingressing mesodermal cells will give rise to the somitic mesoderm.[4,6] The remaining epiblast cells spread out to replace the cells that have ingressed through the primitive groove, forming the ectoderm (both neuroectoderm and surface ectoderm).

The cranial extension of the primitive streak is a specialized structure referred to as Hensen's node. The caudal extension of the primitive streak is referred to as the primitive pit (**Fig. 1–4B**). As the primitive streak regresses, mesodermal cells from Hensen's node ingress through the primitive pit to form the midline notochord (**Fig. 1–4B**).[4,6,7] The notochord continues to elongate as the primitive streak and Hensen's node regress toward the caudal pole of the embryo, and is flanked bilaterally by the newly developed somitic mesoderm. Together, these embryonic tissues will form the axial skeleton (vertebrae and disks). Both the notochord and the somites are laid down in a rostral to caudal direction. The most caudal vertebrae are formed later from somites derived from the caudal cell mass (the remnants of the primitive streak) and from the caudal notochord derived from the posterior notochordal center located immediately cranial to the caudal cell mass.

## Condensation of the Somitic Mesoderm to Form the Somites

Once in its final position the somitic mesoderm aggregates into discrete blocks of tissue, the somites (**Fig. 1–5**); this process appears to be influenced by, but does not require, the presence of the adjacent notochord and neural tube, because somitic mesoderm, when cultured in isolation, is still capable of generating a discrete, segmented pattern.[8,9] In humans, the first somites appear at the beginning of the third embryonic week in the future cervical region.[10] Approximately five cranial somites are present by the time the developing neural tube first begins to close; the formation of succeeding caudal somites keeps pace with the rostral to caudal wave of neurulation.

The patterning of the somites is determined by the interaction of various homeobox genes and their gene products. The specification of a vertebra along the craniocaudal axis is thought to be due to its Hox profile—the degree of expression of various homeobox genes at that particular craniocaudal level. Misexpression of one or another homeobox gene in mice can result in either anterior or posterior transformation of various vertebrae. For example, the overexpression of *Hoxa-7* results in a posterior translocation of the cervical vertebrae such that the last occipital somites, rather than contributing to the occiput, form an aberrant "proatlas." The true atlas, which normally would consist of only a ring and whose cells ordinarily would contribute to the formation of the dens, instead expresses a full vertebral body. In contrast, overexpression of the gene *Hox-6* results in an anterior spinal translocation, creating a thoracic vertebra that has a rib from the upper lumber vertebra.[11] The misexpression of homeobox genes in humans could similarly account for such malformations as the occipitalized atlas, cervical ribs, and lumbarized or sacralized lumbosacral vertebrae.

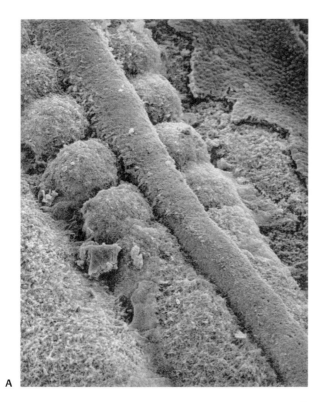

A

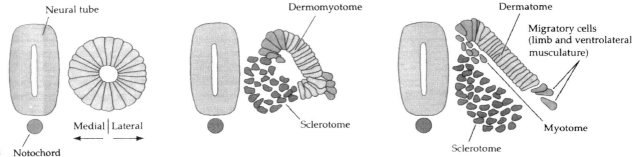

B    Notochord

**Figure 1–5**    Formation of somites. **(A)** Scanning electron micrograph of chick embryo showing the somitic mesoderm forming as blocks of tissue from the unsegmented somitic mesoderm, lying on either side of the midline neural tube.

**(B)** The somite initially forms immediately lateral to the neural tube and notochord. Reorganization within the somite forms the dorsolateral dermomyotome, and the ventromedial sclerotome that will give rise to the vertebrae.

The maximum number of somites in the human embryo is generally given as 42 to 44, although no more than 38 or 39 are required for the formation of the axial skeleton.[10] Most of the "overage" is due to coccygeal somitic segments that disappear during subsequent growth, although a rearrangement or loss of the most cranial segments can occur as well.[12] The number and size of the somites appear to be species specific and relatively constant within species.[13] If somites are experimentally removed, the embryo is capable of compensating (regulating) to generate a normal number of somites of normal size.[14,15] Vertebral malformations of the type seen in clinical practice are rare after experimental excision of somites, suggesting that such malformations may arise later in embryogenesis.

## Formation of the Sclerotome and Dermomyotome

The developing somite becomes reorganized dorsoventrally into two segments: a more ventral sclerotome, which will form the axial skeleton, and a more dorsal dermomyotome, which will form the dermis and subcutaneous tissues of the back as well as the myocytes of the dorsal trunk musculature (**Fig. 1–5**).[9] The sclerotome and dermomyotome are readily identified by the expression of various molecular markers. The sclerotome is characterized by the expression of Pax-1 and Pax-9, whereas the dermomyotome is characterized by the expression of Pax-3 and Pax-7 as well as Myo-D and other molecular species.[16] The formation of the sclerotome and dermomyotome is regulated by the notochord and/or neural tube floor plate (the ventral portion of the neural tube); a dorsally implanted notochord or floor plate represses the formation of the dermomyotome and instead induces an additional sclerotome, whereas the excision of the notochord inhibits formation of the sclerotome ventrally.[9]

The subsequent development of the somites can be divided into three phases: the membranous phase during the fifth week of embryogenesis, the chondrification phase beginning at the sixth embryonic week, and the ossification phase beginning at around the ninth embryonic week.

## Formation of the Membranous Somite and Resegmentation

The membranous phase begins during the fifth week of embryogenesis. Sclerotomal cells from each somitic pair migrate toward the midline and surround the notochord ventrally and the neural tube dorsally. The merging of cells from somites on either side of the notochord produces the vertebral centra, which first become visible in human embryos during the fifth week. Each sclerotome is divided into cranial and caudal halves, each having a unique histological appearance and expressing a different set of cellular and molecular markers.[9] This craniocaudal polarity begins during somite formation and is restricted to the sclerotomal portion of the somite.[16] The cranial portion of each sclerotome contains more loosely packed cells, and the caudal portion contains more densely packed cells. Between the cranial and caudal portions lies a hypocellular cleft, called the fissure of von Ebner. The craniocaudal organization of the sclerotome is critical to axonal outgrowth because the outgrowth of spinal nerves at each level of the neuraxis is restricted to the more loosely packed cranial portion of the sclerotome.[8,16] The dorsal vertebral arch appears to be exclusively derived from the caudal, more densely packed, half of the sclerotome.

There has been ongoing debate about whether each sclerotome forms a single vertebral centrum or whether the caudal half (the dense-celled portion) of one sclerotome and the cranial half of the adjacent sclerotome combine to form a single vertebral body, with the hypocellular fissure of von Ebner contributing

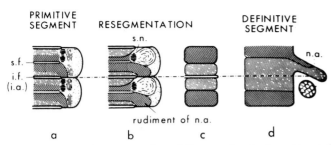

**Figure 1–6** Resegmentation of the somites to form the definitive vertebrae. The densely hatched area is the dense-celled area, the more lightly hatched area the loose-celled area. For details, see text. s.f., segmental fissure (of von Ebner); i.f. and i.a., intersegmental fissure and artery; s.n., ; n.a., neural arch. (Reprinted with permission from Tanaka T, Uhthoff HK. Significance of resegmentation in the pathogenesis of vertebral body malformation. Acta Orthop Scand 1981;52:331–338.)

to the intervening intervertebral disk (a process called resegmentation, or Neugliederung). Resegmentation was originally proposed by Remak[17] in 1855 to account for the anatomical arrangement of the vertebral centra, dorsal vertebral arch, and spinal nerves. Because at each sclerotomal level the spinal nerve passes through the cranial half-sclerotome and the posterior vertebral arch is derived from the caudal half-sclerotome, one would predict that the spinal nerve would exit cranial to the corresponding pedicle. The observation that each spinal nerve passes caudal to the corresponding pedicle could only be accounted for by resegmentation such that the cranial, loose-celled region of one sclerotome would join with the caudal, dense-celled region of the next more cranial sclerotome to form a single vertebral unit (**Fig. 1–6**).

The concept of resegmentation has been opposed by Verbout,[18] Theiler,[19] and others, who have suggested that each vertebra (including the vertebral centrum, posterior arch, transverse processes, ribs, and a single adjacent intervertebral disk) is derived exclusively from a single pair of somites. However, much (but not all) of the experimental evidence supports the concept of resegmentation.[20-22] For example, chick–quail chimeras (in which single chick somites are excised and replaced with quail vertebrae) and retroviral-mediated gene transfer paradigms (in which a recombinant retrovirus expressing a β-galactosidase marker is injected into single somites) have been used to follow the fate of the labeled somite over time. In these experiments, each somite contributes to two adjacent vertebral centra.

## Chondrification Phase

Chondrification centers appear within the sclerotomes during the sixth embryonic week under the inductive control of secreted substances from the adjacent notochord and ventral neural tube. Ordinarily, three paired centers of chondrification appear for each vertebra (**Fig. 1–7**). The first pair surrounds the notochord ventral to the neural tube and forms the vertebral centrum. The second pair forms dorsolaterally and migrates dorsal to the neural tube to form the

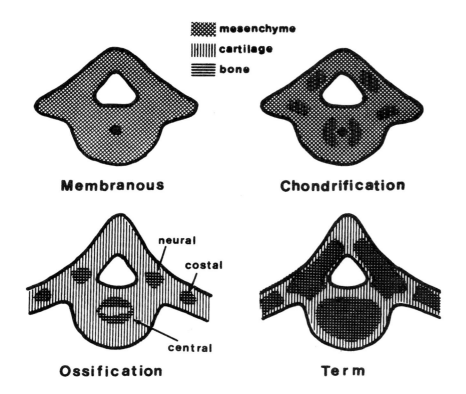

▓▓▓ **mesenchyme**

||||||| **cartilage**

☰ **bone**

**Membranous**          **Chondrification**

**Ossification**          **Term**

neural

costal

central

**Figure 1–7**   Chondrification and ossification of the vertebrae. For details, see text. (Reprinted with permission from Parke WW. Development of the spine. In: Herkowitz HN, Garfin SR, Balderston RA, Eismont FJ, Bell GR, Wiesel SW, eds. Rothman-Simeone The Spine. 4th ed. Philadelphia: WB Saunders; 1999:3–27.)

posterior vertebral arches and spinous processes. The third pair develops between the dorsal and ventral pairs and forms the transverse processes and costal arches. The ventral centers appear earlier than the dorsal centers, resulting in chondrification of the vertebral centra before the dorsal arches. Chondrification begins at the cervicothoracic region and extends both cranially and caudally thereafter. During the chondrification phase, cells from perinotochordal tissues condense around the notochord to produce the anulus of the intervertebral disk, while physaliphorous cells of the notochord form the more centrally located nucleus pulposus.[23] The ALL and PLL are formed during the chondrification phase from mesenchymal cells surrounding the cartilaginous vertebrae.

## Ossification Phase

Ossification of the vertebrae begins during the eighth embryonic week[24] and continues postnatally (**Fig. 1–7**). The number of ossification centers that form within each vertebral segment is still a subject of debate. Most authors suggest the presence of three primary ossification centers—one for the vertebral centrum and one for each side of the dorsal vertebral arch. Within each side of the dorsal arch, the ossification centers extend to form three progressively independent zones of ossification—one each for the pedicles, lamina, and transverse processes. Others have proposed two independent ossification centers within each vertebral centrum—one forming dorsally and the other ventrally—with fusion of the two by the twentieth to twenty-fourth embryonic week. Still others have suggested that as many as six primary ossification centers may be present—two forming the vertebral centrum; two forming the pedicles, lateral masses, and transverse processes; and two forming the laminae and spinous process (reviewed by Ogden et al[23]).

Cartilaginous zones appear cranial and caudal to the ventral ossification centers as the cartilaginous end plates. At the periphery of the cartilaginous end plates, between the developing intervertebral disk and the expanding ossification center of the vertebral centrum, lies the ring apophysis. Because of the ellipsoid growth of the ossification center, the ring apophysis is relatively deficient dorsally and more robust laterally and ventrally, forming a C-shape. By 11 to 14 years postnatally, foci of ossification appear within the ring apophysis, becoming confluent by 15 years of age and forming the radiographic "ring" (the analogue of the secondary ossification centers of long bones).[23] The ring eventually fuses with the vertebral centrum during middle to late adolescence. During childhood, the ring apophysis can fracture, and its fragments can become displaced into the vertebral canal dorsolaterally, where they impinge on nerve roots in the foramina, simulating a herniated intervertebral disk. The junction of the paired posterior and the ventral ossification centers occurs at the neurocentral joint (of Luschka). It is important to recognize that the neurocentral joint lies *within* the vertebral body, not at the junction of the body with the pedicle. The vertebral body is therefore composed of elements derived from both the dorsal and the centrum ossification centers, and the terms *centrum* and *vertebral body* are therefore not strictly synonymous. Secondary ossification centers develop later in embryogenesis and are located in the apophysis (as already described) and the tips of the spinous and transverse processes. The primary and secondary ossification centers fuse by 15 to 16 years of age.

Ossification of the vertebral centra occurs slightly before that of the dorsal arch.[24,25] Ossification of the vertebral centra begins at the thoracolumbar junction from T10 to L1 and rapidly spreads to involve the T2–L4 vertebrae. Thereafter, ossification proceeds in a bidirectional fashion to involve progressively more cranial and caudal vertebrae. In contrast, ossification of the dorsal arches begins simultaneously from C1 to L1 and proceeds in a craniocaudal direction. All ossification centers are visible by 14 weeks' gestation.[24,25]

The notochord continues to contribute cells to the intervertebral disks during the fetal period and the first few years of postnatal life. During the embryonic period, the notochord develops undulations, the first hint of segmentation. At the level of the intervertebral disks, the notochord assumes a more vacuolated appearance, and the intervening portions are stretched into a "mucoid streak" that eventually begins to disappear as ossification centers appear in the adjacent centra. The remaining physaliphorous cells form the nucleus pulposus of the intervertebral disks; occasional microscopic rests may also be found within the vertebral bodies. By the age of 5 years, the proliferation of physaliphorous cells has largely ceased, and usually no viable cells remain in the disk; however, persistent notochordal rests have been found, particularly in incarcerated disks of the sacrum, and likely account for the sacral chordoma.[12]

## ◆ Embryology of the Craniovertebral Junction

Understanding the development of the subaxial spine allows one to understand the complex development of the CVJ. The development of the CVJ is much more complex and embryologically unstable than that of the subaxial spine and leads to unique malformations in this region. The CVJ develops from the four occipital sclerotomes (formed from somite pairs 1–4), and the first and second cervical sclerotomes (formed from somites 5 and 6) (**Fig. 1–8**). The occipital bone, clivus, and occipital condyles are formed from the four occipital sclerotomes (somites 1–4), with sclerotome 4 forming the condyles and paracondylar processes as well as the ring of the foramen magnum. The anterior arch of the atlas is derived from a dense band of tissue, the hypochordal bow (an analogue of the holocentrus vertebra in more primitive species) derived from the fourth occipital sclerotome (somite 4). The posterior arch of the atlas is derived from contributions from the fourth occipital (somite 4) as well as the first cervical (somite 5) sclerotomes. The anterior arch of the atlas is nonossified in 80% of newborn infants and usually ossifies between 6 and 24 months postnatally.[23] The apical, cruciate, and alar ligaments are also derived from the fourth occipital sclerotome.

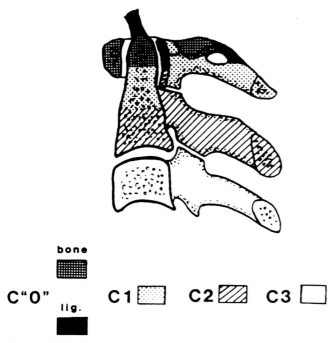

**Figure 1–8**   Development of the craniovertebral junction from the fourth occipital (C" O") and first three cervical (C1,C2,C3). For details, see text. (Reprinted with permission from Parke WW. Development of the spine. In: Herkowitz HN, Garfin SR, Balderston RA, Eismont FJ, Bell GR, Wiesel SW, eds. Rothman-Simeone sclerotomes, The Spine. 4th ed. Philadelphia: WB Saunders; 1999:3–27.)

The axis is derived from the fourth occipital sclerotome (somite 4) and the first and second cervical sclerotomes (somites 5 and 6). Rather than forming the centrum of the atlas, the ventral portion of the first cervical sclerotome (somite 5) instead forms most of the odontoid process. Remnants of the notochord can be found within the odontoid process at the level of the atlas arch, confirming its origin from the centrum.[12] The odontoid process separates from the atlas between the sixth and seventh weeks of gestation. The rostral tip of the odontoid (the phylogenetic equivalent of the proatlas in reptile and avian species) is formed from the fourth occipital sclerotome (somite 4). The remainder of the axis (both the body and dorsal vertebral arch) is derived from the second cervical sclerotome (somite 6).

New information has shed light on the importance of the chondrification stage of CVJ development. Using human embryos, David et al[26] reported that chondrification of the components of the CVJ can be detected as early as 45 days postconception and that the cartilaginous anterior arch of C1 appears at ~50 to 53 days. O'Rahilly and colleagues[27] have described three parts to the cartilaginous odontoid in human embryos of 8 weeks gestation, which they have labeled X, Y, and Z. Parts X and Y correspond to the future odontoid process and part Z to the axis body. The junction of parts X and Y can occasionally be seen as a lobulation in the midportion of the odontoid on lateral roentgenograms in infancy or early childhood.

Ossification of the axis occurs from six ossification centers. The dens contains a bilaterally symmetrical pair of ossification centers that may not fuse until 3 months postnatally.[23] The tip of the dens (the portion derived from the fourth occipital sclerotome) contains an additional ossification center. Finally, the axis body contains three ossification centers—a ventral ossification center forming the centrum and bilaterally paired dorsal ossification centers forming the dorsal arch. Fusion of the dens to the axis body at the dentocentral synchondrosis begins at ~4 years of age and is completed by 8 years; fusion of the apex of the dens to the dens proper occurs at around 12 years.

## ◆ Malformations of the Spine

With the foregoing background, it is now appropriate to discuss malformations of the spine. Although some of these malformations are described in the context of thoracic or lumbosacral locations where they most commonly occur, they provide good examples that illustrate embryogenetic concepts regardless of location and are useful in our discussion of cervical spine malformations. Several classification schemes for spinal malformations have been proposed. The most recent and comprehensive classification by Tsou and colleagues (**Fig. 1–9**) is based on alleged embryogenetic mechanisms[28] and has been modified in response to more recent embryonic data obtained by Tanaka and Uhthoff.[29] These schemes propose that most vertebral malformations arise during the membranous (resegmentation) or early chondrification phases of vertebral

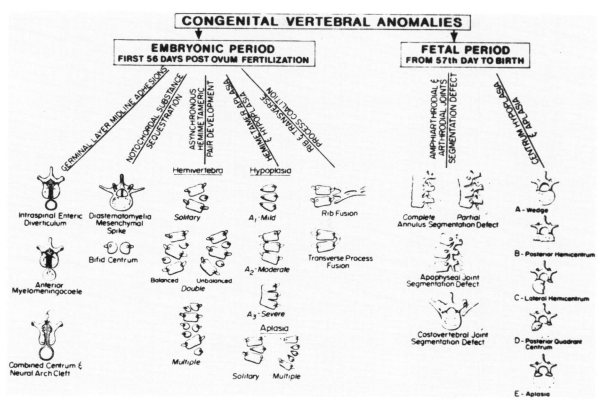

**Figure 1–9**  Proposed schematic of vertebral malformations. For details, see text. (Reprinted with permission from Tsou PM, Yau A, Hodgson AR. Embryogenesis and prenatal development of congenital vertebral anomalies and their classification. Clin Orthop 1980;152:211–231.)

formation, although certain malformations may arise later, during the ossification phase.[28,29] Based on this classification scheme and subsequent modifications, we can divide vertebral malformations into at least seven categories according to reputed embryogenetic mechanism(s), although more than one mechanism may account for each malformation: (1) abnormalities of gastrulation (vertebral anomalies associated with split cord and other complex dysraphic spinal cord malformations); (2) disordered alignment of sclerotomal rests giving rise to hemimetameric shifts (hemivertebrae); (3) disordered formation of whole vertebrae (single or multiple) or of vertebral elements from sclerotomal precursors (vertebral wedging, hemivertebrae, caudal agenesis); (4) disordered segmentation of vertebrae, with or without associated vertebral formation defects [block vertebrae; Klippel-Feil syndrome (KFS)]; (5) disordered alignment of vertebrae (congenital vertebral dislocation); (6) disordered assimilation of sclerotomal cells across the midline (butterfly vertebrae); and (7) disordered ossification and fetal growth (isolated defects of vertebral centra, dysplastic spondylolysis). Although this list is not intended to be comprehensive, the following sections give concrete examples to illustrate the various vertebral malformations and place them into the context of disordered embryogenesis.

Neither the cellular nor the molecular mechanisms underlying these malformations are understood.

## Disordered Gastrulation

Dias and Walker have proposed that certain malformations of the neuraxis and axial skeleton involving tissues derived from all three primary germ cell layers, including split cord and other "complex dysraphic malformations," represent disorders of gastrulation.[30] According to this theory, disordered midline axial integration during the period of primitive streak regression could result in paired notochordal processes and neural tubes (**Fig. 1–10**). Subsequent embryonic repair of this initial disturbance could result in a variety of malformations that, although phenotypically different, share a common embryonic mechanism. In addition to multiple anomalies of the neural tube and other organ systems, a variety of vertebral malformations may arise from the effect of this disturbance on the prospective somitic mesoderm in the proximal half of the primitive streak during gastrulation.[30] Hemivertebrae, sagittally clefted (butterfly) vertebrae, fused (block) vertebrae, midline osseous or fibrocartilaginous spurs or bands, and some types of the Klippel-Feil anomaly, iniencephaly, and sacral agenesis have all been described (reviewed by Dias and Walker[30]). The association of these vertebral malformations with elements of the split cord malformation and its sequelae is the key to identifying this embryopathy.

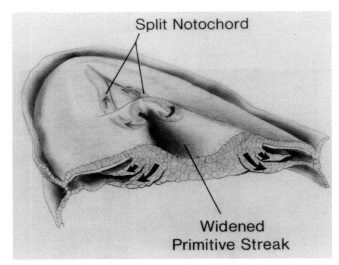

**Figure 1–10**  Proposed embryogenesis of split cord malformations and other "complex dysraphic malformations." Abnormal gastrulation results in a failure of midline axial integration. The primitive streak is abnormally wide; prospective notochordal cells therefore begin ingressing more laterally than normal. As a result, two notochordal processes are formed. The caudal neuroepithelium flanking the primitive streak also fails to become integrated to form a single neuroepithelial sheet, and instead forms two "hemineural plates." The displaced somites (not yet formed) will form abnormal vertebrae. (Reprinted with permission from Dias MS, Walker ML. The embryogenesis of complex dysraphic malformations: a disorder of gastrulation? Pediatr Neurosurg 1992; 18:229–253.)

## Malalignment of Somitic Columns—Hemimetameric Shift

Lehman-Facius[31] first suggested in 1925 that hemivertebrae may arise as a result of a "hemimetameric shift" of the somitic column on one side of the embryo. Tsou et al[28] have argued that, during the integration of the somitic mesoderm across the midline to form individual centra, the somites are normally at the same stage of development and integration occurs between bilaterally juxtaposed pairs of somites. However, tardy development of a somite on one side might lead to a caudal metameric (segmental) shift of one somitic column with respect to the other, malalignment of the somites, and the creation of an unpaired sclerotomic center leading to a hemivertebra (**Fig. 1–10**). The key characteristic of this malformation is a hemivertebral segment that has a rounded medial border and *does not cross the midline.* Both the portion of the vertebral centrum and the corresponding dorsal vertebral arch on the opposite side are congenitally absent.[28] A fully formed posterior vertebral arch is present on the ipsilateral side but is often incorporated into the vertebral arch above or below the hemivertebra and may be difficult to see. The malformation may be uni- or multisegmental and may lead to balanced or imbalanced hemivertebrae. Tsou et al[28] estimate that this mechanism accounts for the majority of cases of hemivertebra (58 of 63 cases in their series).

## Disordered Vertebral Formation

Disruption or injury to the somitic mesoderm during gastrulation, to the somites during segmentation, or to the sclerotomal precursors during the membranous phase could unilaterally decrease the ability of the sclerotome to contribute cells to the formation of the vertebra, resulting in unilateral vertebral hypoplasia or agenesis. Although a disorder of the ossification phase was originally proposed by Junghanns,[32] the presence of these malformations in embryos of 7 to $11^{1}/_{2}$ weeks gestation[29,33] clearly refutes such a mechanism; ossification is likely affected only secondarily. Examples of partially disordered vertebral formation are wedge vertebrae and some cases of hemivertebrae. Tsou et al have applied the term *hemimetameric hypoplasia* or *aplasia* to these malformations, and identify three types related to the severity of the deficiency.[28] A key component is the involvement of both the vertebral centrum and the posterior vertebral arch.

In the mildest form, the quantity of chondrogenic precursors from the ipsilateral sclerotome is reduced, the height of the vertebral centrum is diminished unilaterally, and a wedge vertebra results (**Fig. 1–11**). In the moderate form, the contributions to the posterior vertebral arch are deficient, and the laminae, apophyseal joints, and (in more severe forms) pedicles of adjacent segments fuse to form a dorsolateral unsegmented bar. In the thoracic region, multiple rib malformations are also formed (**Fig. 1–11**). In the most severe form, the vertebral centrum and dorsal arch are simultaneously affected, leading to a form of hemivertebra. In contrast to the hemivertebra formed by hemimetameric shift as already described, however, the existing contralateral half centrum in this instance is irregular and crosses the midline to a variable degree; a rudimentary rib may mark the site of the missing half centrum. In

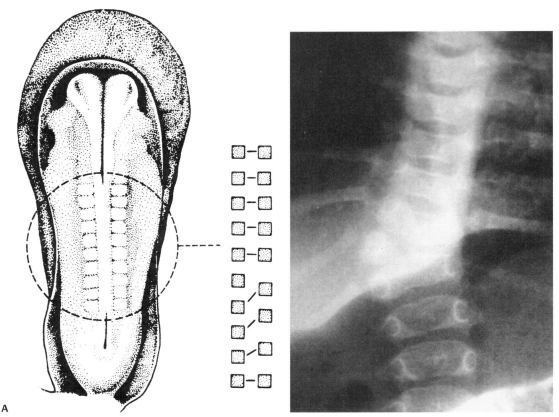

**A**

**B**

**Figure 1–11**    Hemivertebra. **(A)** Schematic illustration of hemimetameric somitic shift producing a hemivertebra. If paired somites are not at the same stage of maturation at the time of somitic midline fusion, the tardy side shifts one segment caudad, producing an isolated hemisomite, which develops into a solitary hemivertebra. (Reprinted with permission from Tsou PM, Yau A, Hodgson AR. Embryogenesis and prenatal development of congenital vertebral anomalies and their classification. Clin Orthop 1980;152:211–231.) **(B)** Anteroposterior radiograph of a hemivertebra.

the extreme, multisegmental failure can occur, and the hemivertebral elements are replaced at multiple levels with poorly differentiated fibrocartilaginous tissue.[28]

Several dysraphic anomalies, most commonly split cord and related malformations, have been associated with hemivertebrae of this type. The combination of a single hemivertebra with a contralateral congenital dorsolateral unsegmented bar is most frequently (50% of cases) associated with an underlying spinal cord malformation.[34] Associated renal malformations are also common, particularly with lower thoracic and lumbar lesions, and are predicted embryologically by the close physical and temporal proximity of the embryonic intermediate mesoderm, which lies lateral to the somitic mesoderm during embryogenesis and which gives rise to the mesonephros of the kidney. When renal malformations coexist with hemivertebrae, they are always ipsilateral to the side of the missing half-vertebra.[35] The underlying cause of the disruption is unknown, although a vascular etiology attributable to malformation or disruption of the intersegmental arteries during the membranous phase has been proposed by Tanaka and Uhthoff.[33] Those associated with dysraphic malformations may arise prior to neural tube closure and involve a disorder of gastrulation as already discussed.[30]

## Disordered Vertebral Segmentation

Several malformations can be ascribed to disorders of vertebral segmentation. The simplest example of isolated failure of vertebral segmentation would be the single block vertebra involving fusion of two adjacent vertebrae. These may be ventral (affecting only the vertebral body), dorsal (affecting only the dorsal vertebral arch), or both. An example of a more restricted dorsolateral failure would be the unsegmented bar (discussed earlier). Multiple vertebral fusions may be involved in the KFS.

The simplest mechanistic explanation would be a failure (within either the prospective somitic mesoderm or the somites themselves) to properly segment into discrete entities, perhaps because of disordered expression of homeobox genes, cell adhesion molecules, or other molecular species. Segmentation appears to be regulated by metameric segmentation genes of the homeobox class and others, and genetic mutations of these genes may be responsible for segmentation failure malformations. Keynes and Stern[8] have described "segmentation-class" gene mutations in mice that display a variety of vertebral fusions, deletions, and malformations. For example, in the mouse mutant *pudgy*, only rudimentary segmentation takes place, resulting in multiple segmentation anomalies and irregular, misshapen vertebrae.[11] Homologues of the *Drosophila* genes *Delta* and *Notch* appear to be particularly important in somite segmentation;[9] mouse mutants lacking in *Notch* expression exhibit severe defects of somitic segmentation and polarity, and microinjections of a dominant negative form of *X-Delta-2* into *Xenopus* embryos cause multiple disorders of segmentation and even abolish the segmental pattern. Whether the localized segmentation failures of block vertebrae are due to these or other mechanisms is unknown.

Alternatively, Tsou et al[28] suggested that osseous metaplasia of the anulus ventrally or the apophyseal or costovertebral joints dorsally during the ossification phase could account for vertebral fusions. Descriptions of human embryos with vertebral fusions as early as 5 to $7^1/_2$ weeks, however, suggest that these malformations occur much earlier, during or before the membranous phase, and reflect an earlier embryonic insult.[29,33] Others have suggested that the cervical vertebral fusions seen in the KFS may reflect a disruption in either or both the subclavian and vertebral artery blood supply to the involved structures at or shortly before the sixth embryonic week. This disruption would give rise not only to the cervical vertebral fusions but also to the Sprengel's deformity, hypoplastic pectoralis muscles, breast hypoplasia, and terminal limb defects that are sometimes associated with KFS.[36,37] However, vascular mechanisms fail to explain the rare associated thoracolumbar or lumbar fusions (KFS type III) and sacral agenesis (KFS type IV).[38] Finally, the reported association of KFS with split cord malformations[30,39] raises the possibility, as reviewed earlier, that certain cases of KFS may arise through disordered midline axial integration during gastrulation.

## Disordered Vertebral Alignment

A rare condition referred to as congenital vertebral dislocation may represent an example of malalignment of vertebrae during early vertebral development. Congenital vertebral dislocation (**Fig. 1–12**) involves a complete vertebral spondyloptosis at a single vertebral level (most commonly at or near the thoracolumbar junction). The more inferior vertebrae are aligned, as are the more superior vertebrae, suggesting that the entire vertebral column has been translocated at a single vertebral level. The spinal canal at the involved level is widened; the pedicles of the more superior vertebra are peculiarly elongated (**Fig. 1–12**), and the dorsal vertebral arch is often dysraphic as well. The spinal cord is intact across the lesion but is almost always low lying (suggesting spinal cord tethering). Despite the severe disruption of the vertebral canal these patients often have few or no neurological deficits. There are few associated malformations, but reported instances of tracheoesophageal fistula and unilateral renal agenesis suggest an early embryonic insult. Dias has proposed that

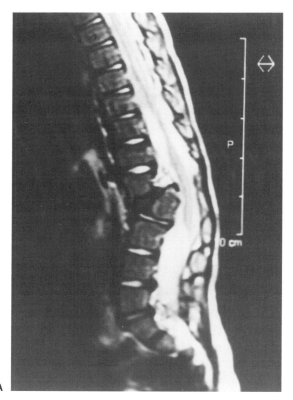

A

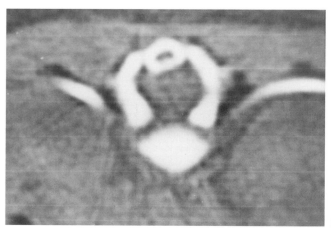

B

**Figure 1–12** Congenital vertebral dislocation. **(A)** T2-weighted sagittal magnetic resonance imaging scan demonstrates a complete and abrupt spondyloptosis of T11 on T12. Note the alignment of the T12 body with the more caudal vertebral column. **(B)** Axial computed tomographic myelogram in another case shows the spinal cord and thecal sac transposed dorsally to the extreme dorsal portion of the spinal canal . The pedicles are abnormally elongated and the canal very widened in the anteroposterior dimension. (Reprinted with permission from Dias MS, Li V, Landi M, Schwend R, Grabb P. The embryogenesis of congenital vertebral dislocation: early embryonic buckling? Pediatr Neurosurg 1998;29:281–289.)

tion with other vertebral malformations. Recent attention has focused on the *Hox* genes, particularly the *Hox* gene *Cdx1* in mice. This gene is expressed in the caudal primitive streak during gastrulation and extends as far rostrally as the caudal hindbrain. Inactivation of *Cdx1* results in anterior homeotic transformation of the vertebrae—the anterior arch of the atlas is fused with the occiput, the posterior arch is hypoplastic, the second and third vertebrae are malformed, and scattered malformations are found as far caudal as the ninth thoracic vertebra. Disruptions of *Hoxb-4* lead to homeotic transformation of the atlas to the axis, whereas disruption of *Hoxd-3* leads to rostral homeotic transformations of both C1 and C2. These experiments suggest an important role of *Hox* genes and their gene products in both the proper specification and segmentation of various craniocervical junction elements.[47]

Incomplete chondrification or ossification could give rise to several malformations. For example, incomplete formation of atlantal chondrification or ossification centers could lead to hypoplasia/aplasia of one or both posterior atlas arches. On the other hand, midline posterior atlantal defects generally are thought to represent a failure of chondrification because the midline defect is filled with connective tissue rather than cartilage.[48]

Abnormal fusion of adjacent ossification centers at the CVJ may produce several well-known malformations. Within the atlas or axis, a failure of anterior and posterior ossification centers to fuse properly will produce characteristic defects involving the predictable sites of normal fusion—anterolaterally and at the posterior midline. A failure of midline fusion between the paired odontoid ossification centers results in a bifid odontoid process. In an analogous manner, a failure of fusion between the ossiculum terminale (fourth cervical sclerotome) and the odontoid process (first cervical sclerotome) results in ossiculum terminale (or os avis); in some cases the ossiculum terminale fuses instead with the distal clivus.

The genesis of the OO is a particularly fascinating study in the embryology of the CVJ. Both traumatic and congenital forms have been proposed. Several illustrative cases in which OO developed months or years following trauma with previously documented radiographs showing a normal odontoid support the view that at least some forms of OO represent posttraumatic pseudarthroses.[49] Others seem more clearly to be congenital in origin. The original embryogenetic theory to explain OO proposed a failure of fusion between the first and second cervical sclerotomes (somites 5 and 6). In a more recent study, however, Currarino et al suggest an alternative mechanism.[50] A close inspection of radiographs in 10 patients with OO revealed that all had defects in the midportion of the odontoid (that is, within the odontoid proper) rather than at the synchondrosis between the odontoid and axis base. Six of these patients had various forms of skeletal dysplasia (diastrophic dysplasia, spondyloepiphyseal dysplasia, pseudoachondroplasia, and Larsen's syndrome). Because no transverse segmentation exists in the midportion of the normal odontoid at any time during embryonic life, these findings led Currarino et al to conclude that OO represents an abnormal complete or partial embryonic segmentation within the odontoid itself.[50] They instead proposed that OO arises because of an embryologically abnormal segmentation (complete or partial) of the midportion of the odontoid, between segments X and Y.

## ◆ Conclusion

This chapter identifies and organizes the various congenital vertebral malformations that are seen clinically. Other chapters in this book describe their clinical aspects and surgical management. The developmental origins of many of these malformations cannot be known with certainty, and it is likely that some—perhaps even all—of the current models will eventually be proven wrong. Attempts to attribute these malformations simplistically to one embryogenetic mechanism (e.g., failure of segmentation) are likely to be supplanted by more sophisticated models that involve the interplay of various genes (such as the *Hox* genes) in a complicated "developmental dance." Despite the limitations of our current models, however, the classification of various congenital vertebral malformations according to their reputed embryonic mechanism(s) at least provides a framework upon which to better understand their anatomy and biomechanics. We anxiously await the next contributions to our understanding of this complex subject.

### References

1. Parke WW, Rothman RH, Brown MD. The pharyngovertebral veins: an anatomical rationale for Grisel's syndrome. J Bone Joint Surg Am 1984;66:568–574
2. O'Rahilly R, Mèuller F, Streeter GL. Developmental Stages in Human Embryos: Including a Revision of Streeter's "Horizons" and a Survey of the Carnegie Collection. Washington, DC: Carnegie Institution of Washington; 1987
3. Vakaet L. Some new data concerning the formation of the definitive endoblast in the chick embryo. J Embryol Exp Morphol 1962;10:38–57
4. Rosenquist GC. A radioautographic study of labeled grafts in the chick blastoderm: development from primitive streak stages to stage 12. Contrib Embryol 1966;38(262):71–110
5. Modak SP. Experimental analysis of the origin of the embryonic endoblast in birds [in French]. Rev Suisse Zool 1966;73:877–908
6. Nicolet G. An autoradiographic study of the presumptive fate of the primitive streak in chick embryos [in French]. J Embryol Exp Morphol 1970;23:70–108
7. Nicolet G. Avian gastrulation. Adv Morphog 1971;9:231–262
8. Keynes RJ, Stern CD. Mechanisms of vertebrate segmentation. Development 1988;103:413–429
9. Gossler A, Hrabe de Angelis M. Somitogenesis. Curr Top Dev Biol 1998;38:225–287
10. Muller F, O'Rahilly R. Somitic-vertebral correlation and vertebral levels in the human embryo. Am J Anat 1986;177:3–19
11. Dietrich S, Kessel M. The vertebral column. In: Thorogood P, ed. Embryos, Genes, and Birth Defects. Chichester: John Wiley and Sons; 1997:281–302
12. Parke WW. Development of the spine. In: Herkowitz HN, Garfin SR, Balderston RA, Eismont FJ, Bell GR, Wiesel SW, eds. Rothman-Simeone The Spine. 4th ed. Philadelphia: WB Saunders; 1999:3–27
13. Flint OP, Ede DA, Wilby OK, Proctor J. Control of somite number in normal and amputated mutant mouse embryos: an experimental and a theoretical analysis. J Embryol Exp Morphol 1978;45:189–202

14. Tam PP. The control of somitogenesis in mouse embryos. J Embryol Exp Morphol 1981;65(Suppl):103–128

15. Bagnall KM, Sanders EJ, Higgins SJ, Leam H. The effects of somite removal on vertebral formation in the chick. Anat Embryol (Berl) 1988;178:183–190

16. Christ B, Schmidt C, Huang R, Wilting J, Brand-Saberi B. Segmentation of the vertebrate body. Anat Embryol (Berl) 1998;197:1–8

17. Remak R. Untersuchungen über die Entwicklung der Wirbelthiere. Berlin: Reimer; 1855

18. Verbout AJ. A critical review of the "Neugliederung" concept in relation to the development of the vertebral column. Acta Biotheor 1976;25:219–258

19. Theiler K. Vertebral malformations. Adv Anat Embryol Cell Biol 1988;112:1–99

20. Ewan KB, Everett AW. Evidence for resegmentation in the formation of the vertebral column using the novel approach of retroviral-mediated gene transfer. Exp Cell Res 1992;198:315–320

21. Bagnall KM. The migration and distribution of somite cells after labelling with the carbocyanine dye, Dil: the relationship of this distribution to segmentation in the vertebrate body. Anat Embryol (Berl) 1992;185:317–324

22. Bagnall KM, Higgins SJ, Sanders EJ. The contribution made by cells from a single somite to tissues within a body segment and assessment of their integration with similar cells from adjacent segments. Development 1989;107:931–943

23. Ogden JA, Ganey TM, Sasse J, Neame PJ, Hilbelink DR. Development and maturation of the axial skeleton. In: Weinstein SL, ed. The Pediatric Spine: Principles and Practice. New York: Raven; 1994:3–69

24. Bareggi R, Grill V, Sandrucci MA, et al. Developmental pathways of vertebral centra and neural arches in human embryos and fetuses. Anat Embryol (Berl) 1993;187:139–144

25. Bareggi R, Grill V, Zweyer M, Narducci P, Forabosco A. A quantitative study on the spatial and temporal ossification patterns of vertebral centra and neural arches and their relationship to the fetal age. Anat Anz 1994;176:311–317

26. David K, McLachlan J, Aiton J, et al. Cartilaginous development of the human craniovertebral junction as visualised by a new three-dimensional computer reconstruction technique. J Anat 1998;192(Pt 2):269–277

27. O'Rahilly R, Muller F, Meyer DB. The human vertebral column at the end of the embryonic period proper, I: The column as a whole. J Anat 1980;131:565–528.

28. Tsou PM, Yau A, Hodgson AR. Embryogenesis and prenatal development of congenital vertebral anomalies and their classification. Clin Orthop 1980;152:211–231

29. Tanaka T, Uhthoff HK. The pathogenesis of congenital vertebral malformations: a study based on observations made in 11 human embryos and fetuses. Acta Orthop Scand 1981;52:413–425

30. Dias MS, Walker ML. The embryogenesis of complex dysraphic malformations: a disorder of gastrulation? Pediatr Neurosurg 1992;18:229–253

31. Lehmann-Facius H. Die Keilwirbelbildung bei der kongenitalen Skoliose. Frankfurter Z. Pathol 1925;31:389

32. Junghanns H. Die Fehlbildungen der Wirbelkörper. Arch Orthop Unfallchir 1937;38:1–24

33. Tanaka T, Uhthoff HK. Significance of resegmentation in the pathogenesis of vertebral body malformation. Acta Orthop Scand 1981;52:331–338

34. McMaster MJ. Congenital scoliosis. In: Weinstein SL, ed. The Pediatric Spine: Principles and Practice. New York: Raven; 1994:227–244

**35.** Tori JA, Dickson JH. Association of congenital anomalies of the spine and kidneys. Clin Orthop 1980;148:259–262

**36.** Bavinck JN, Weaver DD. Subclavian artery supply disruption sequence: hypothesis of a vascular etiology for Poland, Klippel-Feil, and Mobius anomalies. Am J Med Genet 1986;23:903–918

**37.** Brill CB, Peyster RG, Keller MS, Galtman L. Isolation of the right subclavian artery with subclavian steal in a child with Klippel-Feil anomaly: an example of the subclavian artery supply disruption sequence. Am J Med Genet 1987;26:933–940

**38.** Raas-Rothschild A, Goodman RM, Grunbaum M, Berger I, Mimouni M. Klippel-Feil anomaly with sacral agenesis: an additional subtype, type IV. J Craniofac Genet Dev Biol 1988;8:297–301

**39.** David KM, Copp AJ, Stevens JM, Hayward RD, Crockard HA. Split cervical spinal cord with Klippel-Feil syndrome: seven cases. Brain 1996;119(Pt 6):1859–1872

**40.** Dias MS, Li V, Landi M, Schwend R, Grabb P. The embryogenesis of congenital vertebral dislocation: early embryonic buckling? Pediatr Neurosurg 1998;29:281–289

**41.** Ehrenhaft JL. Development of the vertebral column as related to certain congenital and pathological changes. Surg Gynecol Obstet 1943;76:282–292

**42.** Muller F, O'Rahilly R, Benson DR. The early origin of vertebral anomalies, as illustrated by a "butterfly vertebra." J Anat 1986;149:157–169

**43.** Dubousset J. Torticollis in children caused by congenital anomalies of the atlas. J Bone Joint Surg Am 1986;68:178–188

**44.** Saltzman CL, Hensinger RN, Blane CE, Phillips WA. Familial cervical dysplasia. J Bone Joint Surg Am 1991;73:163–171

**45.** Nicholson JT, Sherk HH. Anomalies of the occipitocervical articulation. J Bone Joint Surg Am 1968;50:295–304

**46.** Taitz C. Bony observations of some morphological variations and anomalies of the craniovertebral region. Clin Anat 2000;13:354–360

**47.** Subramanian V, Meyer BI, Gruss P. Disruption of the murine homeobox gene *Cdx1* affects axial skeletal identities by altering the mesodermal expression domains of *Hox* genes. Cell 1995;83:641–653

**48.** Hierholzer J, Isalberti M, Hosten N, Stroszczynski C, Gandini G, Felix R. A rare, complex developmental anomaly of the atlas: embryological and radiological considerations. Neuroradiology 1999;41:901–903

**49.** Ryken T, Menezes A. Cervicomedullary compression in achondroplasia. J Neurosurg 1994;81:43–48

**50.** Currarino G, Rollins N, Diehl JT. Congenital defects of the posterior arch of the atlas: a report of seven cases including an affected mother and son. AJNR Am J Neuroradiol 1994;15:249–254

# 2

# Clinical Biomechanics of the Pediatric Craniocervical Junction and Subaxial Spine

Marcus L. Ware, Nalin Gupta,
Peter P. Sun, and Douglas L. Brockmeyer

Spinal biomechanics is the study of the consequences of external physiological or pathological forces applied to the spinal column.[1] The most important clinical concept regarding the biomechanics of the spine is that of stability. According to White and Panjabi,[2] instability is defined as the "loss of the ability of the spine under physiologic loads to maintain its pattern of displacement so that there is no initial or additional neurological deficit, no major deformity, and no incapacitating pain." This definition allows the clinician to make interpretations based on the initial injury as well as the known natural history of certain injuries and conditions. This definition also allows certain spinal deformities to be considered stable as long as they do not lead to neurological insult or incapacitating pain. The body of knowledge used to classify injuries as stable or unstable is gathered by anatomical studies, radiographic studies, and mechanical loading experiments on cadavers.

Most of the studies of biomechanics of the cervical spine have focused on adults. Conceptual simplifications with models such as the two-column and three-column spine are created to make predictions as to whether a specific injury pattern is unstable.[3–6] Although pediatric cadavers are rare, it is clear from clinical experience that the pediatric spine is not a scaled down adult spine and has unique biomechanical considerations with different patterns of injuries and different criteria for spinal instability. Furthermore, the unique and complex articulations of the craniocervical junction render modeling extremely difficult. Models created for the subaxial spine do not apply to the craniocervical junction. Many assumptions about the biomechanics of the pediatric craniocervical junction are, therefore, derived from clinical data and extrapolated biomechanical studies from the adult spine. Criteria for clinical instability have relied on a host of radiographic measurements of the various bony landmarks in the occipitoatlantoaxial (O–C2) complex. This chapter reviews the anatomy of the craniocervical junction and discusses the elements involved in maintaining the stability of the O–C2 complex. Also reviewed are the anatomy of the subaxial spine and the elements involved in maintaining stability of the subaxial spine.

## ◆ Review of Normal Biomechanics

### Craniocervical Junction: Normal Kinematics

The biomechanical unit of the craniocervical junction is the occipitoatlantoaxial (O–C2) complex. The occipitoatlantal (O–C1) joint and the atlantoaxial (C1–C2) joint of the O–C2 complex function together as a single unit that controls the movement of the head in relation to the spine. Within this unit, the atlas (C1) serves as a wedged washer between two spheres of mobility (**Fig. 2–1**). The articulation between the occipital condyles and the atlas is cup shaped in the sagittal plane and medially tilted in the coronal plane. This orientation allows up to 20 degrees of flexion/extension and 8 degrees of lateral bending.[2] Flexion and extension at O–C1 is ultimately limited by the contact of the rim of the cup-shaped atlas against the base of the skull.[7] Lateral rotation beyond 8 degrees is restrained by the physiological separation limit of the contralateral O–C1 joint. Rotation at the O–C1 joint is largely blocked by the oblique bony alignment of the articulation. Whereas classic cadaver studies have shown an absence of rotation between the occiput and C1, more recent in vivo studies have shown up to 4 degrees of axial rotation to one side between O and C1.[8,9] In contrast, the biconvex cartilage articulating surface and laterally tilted facet orientation between the atlas and axis allow a large degree of rotation centered about the dens. Up to 60% of the axial rotation of the entire cervical spine occurs at C1–C2, with a described range of 32.2 to 47 degrees to one side.[10-12] Kinking and stretching of the vertebral artery have been described at the transverse foramina after 30 degrees of rotation at the ipsilateral artery and after 45 degrees of rotation at the contralateral artery.[13,14] Sagittal movement of the arch of the atlas along the slightly dorsally curved dens provides additional flexion and extension of 20 degrees at C1–C2. Very little lateral bending occurs at C1–C2.

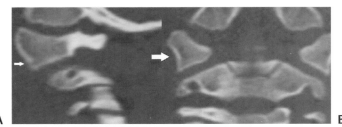

A                                                                B

**Figure 2–1** **(A)** Sagittal reconstruction of a computed tomographic (CT) image of C1 through its lateral mass in a normal child. The arrow is pointing to the lateral mass of C1. **(B)** Coronal reconstruction of a CT scan of C1 in the same patient. The arrow is pointing to the lateral mass of C1.

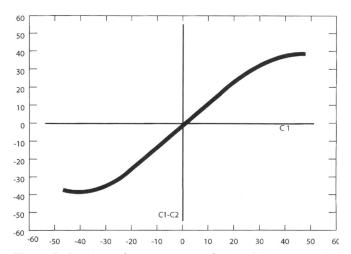

**Figure 2–2**   Normal motion curve of C1 and C2 rotation (Adapted from Pang D, Sun PP. Pediatric vertebral column and spinal cord injuries. In: Youmans JR, ed. Neurological Surgery. Philadelphia: WB Saunders; 2004:3515–3557).

The dynamics of axial rotation can be described by a motion curve where the degrees of rotation are plotted on an x- and y-axis (**Fig. 2–2**). Because there is minimal rotation at O–C1, the head essentially moves with C1 during rotation, and the degree of head axial rotation is essentially the same as the degree of C1 rotation. This is plotted on the x-axis. The degree of rotation between C1 and C2 is plotted on the y-axis. In vivo data on the motion of C1 on C2 has been obtained by computed tomography (CT) and magnetic resonance imaging (MRI).[8,10] The motion curve starts off linear for the first 20 to 30 degrees of rotation because C1 initially moves entirely independently of C2 and the degree of rotation of the C1 is the same as the degree of rotation between C1 and C2. This means that the initial phase of head rotation—the first 20 to 30 degrees—occurs at the C1–C2 joint. As the articular joint capsules and alar ligaments become taut, C2 begins to follow C1 in rotation, and the motion curve flattens out until the limit of the range of motion is reached between C1 and C2. Subsequent head turning is then allowed by subaxial rotation.

Axial rotation is coupled with motions in other axes in the O–C2 unit. Maximal axial rotation is coupled with 1.7 to 4.9 degrees of lateral bending to the opposite direction at O–C1 and 3 degrees of lateral bending to the opposite direction at C1–C2.[12] Rotation is also coupled to extension: up to 13 degrees at the O–C1 joint and 6 degrees at the C1–C2 joint. Downward translation between C1 and C2 is also seen with rotation, presumably from the biconvexity of the articulations.

## Subaxial Cervical Spine: Normal Kinematics

The stability of the subaxial spine (C2–C7) depends on the ability of the vertebral column and intervertebral disks to withstand compressive forces and on the ability of the ligaments connecting these elements to allow for normal motion while resisting forces that would lead to pathological deformity. The intrinsic biomechanical properties of the vertebral bodies and geometric considerations are important in determining the ability of the subaxial cervical spine to withstand physiological stressors.

In this region of the spine, the vertebral bodies are aligned directly above one another, separated by intervertebral disks. The opposing surfaces of the vertebral bodies are gently curved in the sagittal plane. Between any two bodies, the anterior-inferior border of the upper body hangs downward toward the anterior-superior surface edge of the vertebra below. The superior surface slopes downward and forward. This shape is conducive to the flexion–extension motion that occurs at this joint. In the adult, the total range of flexion and extension is 60 to 75 degrees. The greatest motion of flexion and extension is at the O–C1 junction (13 degrees), and the next greatest is between C5 and C7. Dynamic radiographs in children show that the upper cervical segments in infants and children are hypermobile in flexion. The fulcrum for maximal flexion is at C2–C3 in infants and young children, at C3–C4 in children ages 5 or 6 years, and at C5–C6 in adolescents and young adults.[14–16] The predilection for C2 and C3 forward displacement occurs because the joint is more mobile in children given that the articular facets of C2 and C3 lie in a relatively horizontal plane allowing for forward displacement. The more caudal cervical facets are more vertical, such that subluxation would require more force.[16]

The vertebral bodies in the subaxial cervical spine are also curved from side to side. The inferior surface of the upper vertebral body is slightly convex posteriorly, and this convexity is received by a concavity of the body below and by its uncinate process. This shape promotes a side-to-side rocking motion.[7] In adults, the facets are directly opposed to each other, and the mature uncinate processes provide additional support and prevent lateral and rotational movements.[7] In children, however, the facet joints are more horizontally oriented and provide less resistance to rocking and translation between vertebrae. In addition, the uncinate processes are absent in children under the age of 10 years.[16,17] The overall orientation and shape of the vertebral bodies in children allow more motion to physiological loads.

The intervertebral disks are located between vertebral bodies and must respond to a variety of load vectors during physiological and traumatic load, including compression, bending, and tension.[18] The intervertebral disks consist of an anteriorly well-developed and thick anulus that tapers laterally and posteriorly. There is no true anulus posteriorly, only a few fibers near the median plane. The thick anterior anulus acts as an interosseus ligament and resists extensions. The nucleus pulposus at birth has a water content of 88% and contributes to the general malleability of the cervical spine. In loading of the cervical spine, the intervertebral disks carry over 60% of the compressive loads.[19]

## Determinants of Stability at the Craniocervical Junction

Stability at the craniocervical junction level is achieved by three structures that provide major elements of support and two structures that provide minor support. The major supporting structures are the cup-shaped joints at the craniocervical articulation, the capsular ligaments, and the tectorial membrane.[20] At the C1–C2 joint, two major structures provide stability.[21] These structures are the odontoid process and the transverse ligament. They provide the majority of stability at the C1–C2 joint, and their integrity is critical. The transverse ligament is a thick horizontal band of the cruciate ligament that attaches to the inner aspect of the C1 ring, and straps hold the dens against the anterior arch of C1. It is the pivotal stabilizer against horizontal translation of the dens into the spinal canal. In adults, the ligament is 7 to 8 mm thick and can withstand 350 N of force.[22] The strength of the transverse ligament is clinically illustrated by the occurrence of dens fractures in adults and synchondrosis failure in young children while the ligament itself remains intact.

Although the transverse ligament holds the C1 ring against the dens, a unique aspect of the O–C2 region is that, unlike the remainder of the spine, stability is otherwise not primarily provided by the segmental structures (**Fig. 2–3**). The loose articular capsules and thin atlantoaxial and occipitoatlantal membranes between the occiput and C1 and between C1 and C2 allow an extensive range of motion but are not the dominant stabilizers.[2] In addition, there is no correlate of the segmental interspinous ligament in the O–C2 region. The posterior interspace between O–C1 and C1–C2 is filled with suboccipital musculature that is attached to the underlying posterior occipitoatlantal and atlantoaxial membrane dural complex. These small and delicate muscles are theorized to have proprioceptive functions but are unlikely to limit motion.[23]

The stability in the O–C2 region is largely provided by the internal ligaments and muscles directly between the occiput and C2. Among the internal ligaments, the tectorial membrane and alar ligaments are especially important, as demonstrated by Werne in a series of cadaver studies.[24] The tectorial membrane is a well-developed continuation of the posterior longitudinal ligament

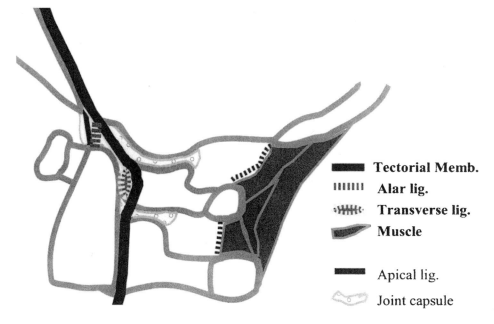

- ▬▬ **Tectorial Memb.**
- ‖‖‖‖ **Alar lig.**
- ⪧╫╫╫⪦ **Transverse lig.**
- ◤ **Muscle**

- ▬▬ **Apical lig.**
- ⬭ Joint capsule

**Figure 2–3** Ligaments of the craniocervical junction. This panel schematically shows the normal ligaments of the craniocervical junction.

(PLL) that holds the body of C2 firmly to the clivus and the anterior rim of the foramen magnum. Initial flexion in the occipitoatlantoaxial unit is limited by skeletal contact between the basion and dens. Additional flexion moves the basion forward and downward over the dens. The tectorial membrane limits this movement by draping and stretching over the dens between the basion and the body of the axis. Extension is also checked by the tectorial membrane and by bony contact between the opisthion and the arch of C1. Lateral bending and rotation are controlled by the alar ligaments, which span obliquely from the posterolateral surface of the dens, attach partly to C2, and then attach to the medial occipital condyles. Sectioning of the tectorial membrane alone results in increased range of flexion and extension as well as vertical translation beyond the normal range between the dens and cranium. Removal of the alar ligaments results in increased contralateral bending and rotation. When both the alar ligaments and tectorial membrane are cut, frank occipital subluxation results. In vivo clinical MRI data in children also demonstrate that involvement of the tectorial membrane in O–C2 injuries is a critical threshold for instability. Although there is a spectrum of various traumatic abnormalities of O–C2 ligamentous and muscular structures, clinical manifestations of instability such as spinal cord injury, radiographic dislocation, and posttraumatic deformity occurred only when the tectorial membrane is involved.[25] The remainder of the occipital-–axial connections, namely, the ascending band of cruciate ligament and the apical ligament, are too delicate to limit motion. In fact, the apical ligament has been shown to be a vestigial structure that offers no stability and is absent in 20% of cadavers studied.[26]

Muscular action and bony contact also contribute to the stability of the O–C2 unit. In vitro studies in which the muscles have been removed revealed that the O–C1–C2 complex has a much larger neutral zone than the subaxial spine and that a much smaller load is needed to create a large displacement.[27] The frequent involvement of the muscles in an isolated injury or in consistent association with other ligamentous disruptions in the O–C2 region supports the idea that they also provide considerable stabilization in the craniocervical region.[25] Hence, muscular action is thought to be substantially responsible for holding the cranium firmly to the spine.

## Determinants of Stability of the Subaxial Cervical Spine

Stability within the subaxial spine relies on the ability of vertebral bodies, intervertebral disks, and facet joints to withstand physiological compressive forces and of the spinal ligaments to withstand physiological tensile forces. The cervical spine can withstand substantial compressive loads during physiological conditions. In the adult, the compressive load increases during flexion and extension and is estimated to reach 1200 N in activities involving maximal isometric muscle efforts.[28,29] Biomechanical studies also suggest that neck posture and the direction in which the load is applied are important in determining the ability of the spine to withstand compressive forces.[29,30] As mentioned previously, the pediatric spine is more flexible, and neck musculature is underdeveloped in younger children. Taken together, these data suggest that, for any given compressive load, the pediatric spine is more likely to sustain injury; however, biomechanical studies with pediatric cadavers are needed to better study the ability of the pediatric cervical spine to withstand compressive loads.

The subaxial cervical spine has been classified into anterior and posterior column elements by the combined experience of Holdsworth,[3] Nicoll,[4] and Roaf.[6] The anterior column consists of the anterior longitudinal ligament (ALL), the vertebral body, the PLL, the anterior and posterior half of the anulus fibrosus, and the intertransverse ligaments. The posterior column consists of the pedicles, lamina, transverse process, spinous processes, interspinous ligaments, supraspinous ligaments, ligamenta flava, and capsular ligaments. Early studies in which the ligaments were cut from posterior to anterior in some spines and anterior to posterior in others suggested that if a motion segment has all its anterior elements plus one additional structure or all its posterior elements plus one structure, it will probably remain stable under physiological loads.[31,32] A recent study by Richter et al[33] showed that in the adult cervical spine in vitro, loss of the ALL alone led to statistically significant increases in range of motion. This range of motion was also increased with sectioning of the ALL and anterior anulus fibrosus, sectioning of the ligamenta flava and interspinous and supraspinous ligaments, and capsulotomy of the facet joints. These studies underscore the importance of the cervical ligaments in maintaining stability in the subaxial spine.

## ◆ Special Pediatric Considerations

The craniocervical junction is the most vulnerable area for potential instability in the pediatric cervical spine. The O–C2 articulations are anatomically more unstable in young children. The occipital condyles are smaller and the occipitoatlantal articulation itself is shallower in the sagittal plane and almost horizontal in the coronal plane.[34] Furthermore, the major stabilizing ligaments and musculature are more elastic and less developed. The presence of unfused synchondrosis between the dens and the body of C2 before age 6 offers a potential vulnerability. Fractures of the odontoid in young children almost always occur as an epiphyseal separation of the growth plate.[35] Occult O–C2 congenital anomalies such as os odontoideum and occipitalization of the atlas may render the O–C2 region vulnerable to even relatively minor trauma.

In addition to the anatomical differences of the O–C2 complex itself, the relatively large head and shorter neck of the young child place the fulcrum of the pediatric cervical spine within the O–C2 complex. Children are commonly involved in motor vehicle accidents and falls that involve impacts of either the head or torso. These mechanisms accelerate the head relative to the torso to concentrate disruptive forces at the O–C2 region. As a result, injury of the O–C2 region is the most common cervical spine injury in children under 10 years of age.[36-38] Injuries to the O–C2 region in children are mostly ligamentous or other soft tissue disruptions rather than fractures. The resulting craniocervical dislocation is highly unstable and demands prompt diagnosis for optimal treatment.

Not all injuries in children involve the craniocervical junction and upper cervical spine, however. Some injuries involve the subaxial cervical spine, and these injuries must be considered as well. The inherent mobility of the pediatric subaxial spine allows for considerably more movement at each motion segment in response to loading forces; this is due to several features. First, the spinal ligaments and joint capsules are sufficiently elastic to withstand considerable stretching without tearing.[39] This quality may account for the radiological finding of pseudosubluxation in children. Second, the intervertebral disk and anulus in children are exceedingly expansible in the longitudinal axis and allow for more distraction.[40] Third, the facet joints in children are shallow and oriented more horizontally than in adults, permitting translation as well as flexion and extension movements. Fourth, the immature vertebral bodies are shorter anteriorly, creating a wedge shape so that forward movement of adjacent segments is enhanced. Fifth, the uncinate processes, which restrict lateral and rotational movements between the bodies, are absent in children under 10 years of age. Sixth, the growth zone in the vertebral end plate splits readily from the primary centrum under moderate shear forces. Finally, the disproportionately large size of an infant's head coupled with relatively weak musculature predisposes the infant's neck to wide excursions when the child is subject to flexion and extension forces.

Spinal cord injury without radiographic abnormality (SCIWORA) is an injury type seen in children that is largely dependent on the flexibility of the pediatric spine. SCIWORA, first described as a syndrome by Pang and Wilberger,[41] is most frequently seen in younger children and is associated with a high incidence of more serious neurological injury. Anywhere from 22 to 67% of children with SCIWORA develop neurological deficit in a delayed fashion (up to 2 days) after what may have been considered a minor injury.[41-44] Once initiated, there may be evolution to severe and irreversible neurological injury. The concept of this problem is based on the premise that the elastic juvenile spine can accommodate considerable intersegmental displacement without fractures or ligamentous rupture, but this displacement is significant enough to precipitate significant spinal cord injury. Four mechanisms may be involved in the pathogenesis of SCIWORA: hyperextension, flexion, distraction, and spinal cord ischemia.[45]

Hyperextension of the cervical spine forces the interlaminar ligaments to bulge forward into the spinal canal and may cause up to 50% narrowing of the canal diameter.[46,47] Cadaver studies have shown that violent hyperextension can cause rupture of the ALL, shearing of the intervertebral disks from the end plate, and displacement of the vertebral body into the spinal canal.[47] Dynamic radiography also showed that elastic recoil of the displaced segment could result in spontaneous reduction, leading to a normal radiographic appearance.[48] Intersegmental movement in the pediatric spine is facilitated by the elasticity of the intraspinal ligaments and the horizontally oriented facets. The immature vertebral body splits readily from its end plate within the brittle growth zone and leaves no radiographic trace of fracture. Similar factors predispose children to hyperflexion myelopathy without evidence of bone or ligamentous injury. The elastic elements, horizontal facets, wedge-shaped bodies, and absence of an uncinate process all tend to facilitate forward interbody movement. The pediatric spine is also vulnerable to distraction injury.[49,50] The elastic spinal column of neonatal cadavers could be stretched up to 2 in. without structural damage, whereas the spinal cord ruptures if it is stretched more than 0.25 in.[51] These findings are supported by cases of frank cord rupture with intact vertebral columns in infants who had undergone forceful breech extraction.[16,17,52] Finally, the architecture of the occipitoatlantal articulations predisposes the upper cervical cord to ischemic necrosis from vertebral artery occlusion.

## ◆ Clinical Instability at the Craniocervical Junction

Criteria for evaluating a patient for instability at the craniocervical junction consist of information obtained from several studies. Failure of the transverse ligament renders the O–C2 unit unstable by allowing posterior dislocation of the dens into the spinal canal. As described earlier, the tectorial membrane also appears to be of particular importance: disruption of the tectorial membrane is a critical threshold for the instability of the O–C2 unit. Traumatic abnormalities of these ligaments can be directly visualized with MRI.[25,53]

The major practical consideration to determine instability, however, has been based on plain radiographs (**Fig. 2–4**). The radiographic result of transverse ligament failure is the widening of the atlantodental interval (ADI). Many

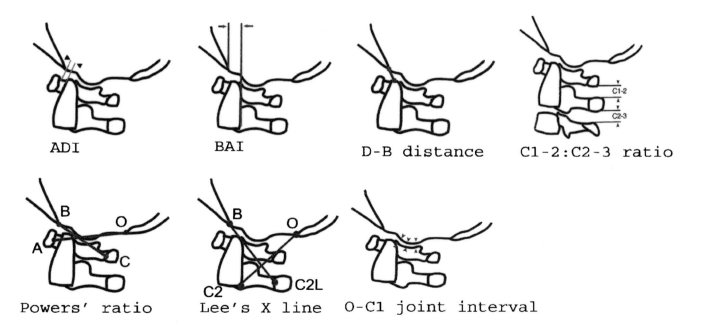

**Figure 2–4** Radiographic assessment of stability. This panel schematically shows the various distances and ratios used to assess plain radiographs for evidence of instability. ADI, atlantodental interval; BAI, basion–axial interval; B, basion; C, posterior arch of atlas; O, opisthion; A, anterior arch of atlas; C2, base of C2; C2L, C2 lamina.

authors accept that the normal upper limit of normal ADI is 3 to 4 mm in adults and 4 mm in children,[13,54] although White and Panjabi accept 5 mm as the upper limit of normal in children.[2] Up to 6 mm of normal separation can be seen in cadaver studies of children less than 10 years of age.[55] When the ADI exceeds 10 mm, the alar ligaments and tectorial membrane may become secondarily damaged from the displaced dens, resulting in O–C1 joint instability as well.[56] In the setting of a C1 ring fracture, if the bilateral overhangs of the lateral masses on the anteroposterior view totals 7 mm or more, a rupture of the transverse ligament should also be suspected.[57]

Additional radiographic criteria have been devised to infer instability at the craniocervical junction. It is important to recognize that once the major stabilizing structures between the occiput and C2 are disrupted in the O–C2 complex and the critical threshold for instability is reached, various displacements between the occiput and C1, between C1 and C2, as well as between the occiput and C2 can be seen. Extrinsic forces of positioning and immobilization in these highly unstable injuries may determine the anatomical relationship of the bony elements postinjury. In children, these forces would tend to be flexion with the relatively larger head size and distraction in a collar.

One criterion for instability is the distance between the dens and basion (DB distance). The upper limit of DB distance is described as 5 mm in adults and between 10 and 12.5 mm in children.[58,59] The variable ossification of the proatlas at the tip of the dens between 2 and 6 years makes application of the DB distance potentially problematic in children. The normal range of sagittal plane translation between the dens and the basion did not dynamically exceed 1 mm in Wiesel and Rothman's study of flexion–extension radiographs in adults.[60] Direct measurements of the O–C1 joint interval on plain films in children by Kaufman et al found that the interval should not exceed 5 mm between any opposing points of the joint articulation.[61] Using CT data, Pang et al described 3 mm as the upper limit of normal for the O–C1 joint interval in children.[45] Harris et al have described the measurement of the basion–axial interval (BAI) as a method to determine the translational relationship between the occiput and C2.[62] The BAI is the distance between the basion and the rostral extension of the posterior cortical margin of the axis (posterior axial line) taken from supine lateral cervical radiographs at age 40. In adults, the BAI normally extends from 12 mm anterior to 4 mm posterior to the posterior axial line. This range does not change with flexion or extension. In 50 children, the BAI was also found to be within 12 mm anterior to the posterior axial line, but the basion did not extend posterior to the posterior axial line.[62] In very young children, however, the posterior cortical margin of the axis is anteriorly sloped, and the BAI may underestimate the degree of anterior occipital translation.

Measurements taken from radiographs are subject to variable magnification from different film target distances. Three measurement methods have been proposed that are dimensionless: the Powers' ratio, the X line, and the C1–C2:C2–C3 ratio.[25,63,64] The Powers' ratio is the distance from the basion to the posterior arch of the atlas (BC) divided by the distance from the opisthion to the anterior arch of the atlas (OA) (**Fig. 2–4**). The BC:OA ratio is 0.77 ± 0.09 in the normal population. All ratios over 1 are abnormal, whereas 150 normal subjects studied by Powers et al[24] had ratios below 0.9. Up to 70% of lateral cervical spine films in children, however, do not reveal the exact position of the opisthion. Anomalies of the posterior arch of C1 and the foramen magnum could make this ratio invalid. Whereas the Powers' ratio requires calculation, the X line proposed by Lee et al[64] does not (**Fig. 2–4**). These investigators drew two lines on the lateral cervical radiograph, the Basion to C2 lamina L and C2 to the opisthion O, which forms an X shape. The Basias to C2 lamina L and C2 opisthion O should tangentially intersect the posterior superior dens and the highest point on the C1 spinolaminar line, respectively. At least one intersection should be present. If the lines fail to intersect, instability should be suspected. This method is seldom applied in the diagnosis of children. Its validity depends on atlantoaxial integrity and a fully developed dens. Finally, because O–C2 instability may be manifest as separation of C1–C2 as well as O–C2, a C1–C2:C2–C3 ratio has been proposed.[25] Ratios greater than 2.5:1 are considered abnormal.

Structural compromise of the bony components in the O–C2 complex can result in instability. In biomechanical studies in adults, resection of greater than 75% of the occipital condyle on one side or an anterior C1 laminectomy with an odontoidectomy results in significant instability.[65] Pure bony injuries such as C2 pedicle fractures that result in instability have been reported in children.[66] Most are stable injuries without neurological deficits. Rigid immobilization is recommended if there is more than 3 mm of displacement of C2 on C3.[67]

## ◆ Clinical Instability of the Subaxial Cervical Spine

The stability of spinal injuries in children, like adults, is dependent on the initial injuries at the time of the trauma and the biomechanical forces acting on the spine after trauma. There are two ways of predicting stability in the cervical spine. The first is to use a simplified model of the subaxial spine as a two- or three-column structure. The second is to make predictions based on the degree of injury and angulation of each level of the spine. As mentioned before, the use of a two-column model to describe subaxial spine stability is derived from the clinical experience of Holdsworth,[3] Nicoll,[4] and Roaf.[68] To review, the major anterior column supporting structures consist of the vertebral body, disk, ALL, and PLL. The major posterior column supporting structures consist of the interspinous and supraspinous ligaments, the ligamenta flava, and the apophyseal joints. The stability of the spine depends largely on the integrity of the posterior ligament complex, and thus injury to the posterior column is considered unstable. In many cases, the two-column model is able to predict spinal stability; however, there are some situations where the two-column model is unable to determine spinal stability accurately. The three-column model of the spine was later described by Denis in categorizing acute thoracolumbar spinal injuries.[5] According to this model, the anterior column consists of the ALL, the anterior anulus, and the anterior wall of the vertebral body. The middle column consists of the PLL, the posterior anulus fibrosus, and the posterior wall of the vertebral body. The posterior column is the same as that in the two-column model. Denis added a "middle" column based on results from experimental studies which suggested that disruption of the entire posterior ligament complex alone is not enough to produce instability. When the PLL and the posterior portion of the anulus are disrupted, the spine becomes unstable. According to this model, loss of integrity of two of the three columns results in instability. Although conceptually simple and readily applicable in clinical situations, the three-column model has limitations. Inclusion of a middle column has a theoretical advantage in thoracic and lumbar injuries, but these considerations are not nearly as important in the cervical region.[69] The pediatric spine is not represented very well by either of these models.

In cases of ligamentous injury, there are often subtle findings on radiographs, and the guidelines for overt instability in children are not well defined. Biomechanical studies in the subaxial spine by White and Panjabi and their associates showed that the angle between adjacent vertebrae in normal adults is always less than 11 degrees and that deformities greater than 11 degrees are considered unstable.[70,71] In children, because the spine is much more elastic and likely to recoil, the upper limit of angulation between adjacent vertebrae that would suggest ligamentous injury is 7 degrees. If a child does not have a neurological deficit and has an angulation greater than 7 degrees but less than 11 degrees, flexion–extension studies should be obtained. If the angulation is unchanged with dynamic study, the study should be repeated in 3 to 5 days to eliminate the effect of spasm. If the angle is again less than 11 degrees and the study is satisfactory (without evidence of spasm), a cervicothoracic brace should be worn for 2 months, after which dynamic radiographs should be obtained to confirm ligamentous healing. If the angulation is less than 7 degrees but the patient has severe pain and spasm, a collar should be worn until dynamic studies can be repeated in a few days to rule out instability.

In addition, White and Panjabi showed that in adults, horizontal interbody displacement of greater than 3.5 mm implies significant ligamentous injury that will result in delayed instability.[2,71] In children, the spine is more flexible, and 3.5 mm of subluxation may be physiological. Thus, in children younger than 8 years, horizontal displacement at the C2–C3 and C3–C4 joints of greater than 4.5 mm should be considered unstable.[72] In children older than 8 years, horizontal displacement greater than 3.5 mm at any level should be considered unstable.

## ◆ Conclusion

The pediatric cervical spine has numerous biomechanical properties that make it significantly different from its adult counterpart. In addition, the forces acting on the pediatric spine under physiological conditions and trauma are different and thus account for the different injury types observed in children. Recent biomechanical studies of the adult spine have greatly advanced our knowledge of the role of individual components of the spine. Similar studies in children are required to improve our understanding of injury patterns in the pediatric spine.

## References

1. Yoganandan N, Pintar F, Maiman DJ, et al. Kinematics of the lumbar spine following pedicle screw plate fixation. Spine 1993;18:504–512
2. White AA, Panjabi MM. Clinical Biomechanics of the Spine. Philadelphia: JB Lippincott; 1990
3. Holdsworth F. Fractures, dislocations, and fracture-dislocations of the spine. J Bone Joint Surg Am 1970;52:1534–1551
4. Nicoll EA. Fractures of the dorso-lumbar spine. J Bone Joint Surg Br 1949;31:376–394
5. Denis F. Spinal instability as defined by the three-column spine concept in acute spinal trauma. Clin Orthop 1984;189:65–76
6. Roaf R. Spinal injuries. Burma Med J 1960;8:139–143
7. Bogduk N, Mercer S. Biomechanics of the cervical spine, I: Normal kinematics. Clin Biomech (Bristol, Avon) 2000;15:633–648
8. Ishii T, Mukai Y, Hosono N, et al. Kinematics of the upper cervical spine in rotation: in vivo three-dimensional analysis. Spine 2004;29:E139–E144
9. Iai H, Goto S, Yamagata M, et al. Three-dimensional motion of the upper cervical spine in rheumatoid arthritis. Spine 1994;19:272–276
10. Dvorak J, Panjabi MM. Functional anatomy of the alar ligaments. Spine 1987;12:183–189
11. Panjabi M, Dvorak J, Duranceau J, et al. Three-dimensional movements of the upper cervical spine. Spine 1988;13:726–730
12. Iai H, Moriya H, Goto S, Takahashi K, Yamagata M, Tamaki T. Three-dimensional motion analysis of the upper cervical spine during axial rotation. Spine 1993;18:2388–2392
13. Fielding JW. Cineroentgenography of the normal cervical spine. J Bone Joint Surg Am 1957;39-A:1280–1288
14. Braakman R, Penning L. The hyperflexion sprain of the cervical spine. Radiol Clin Biol 1968;37:309–320
15. Baker DH, Berdon WE. Special trauma problems in children. Radiol Clin North Am 1966;4:289–305
16. Townsend EH Jr, Rowe ML. Mobility of the upper cervical spine in health and disease. Pediatrics 1952;10:567–574
17. Bailey DK. The normal cervical spine in infants and children. Radiology 1952;59:712–719
18. Matsunaga S, Kabayama S, Yamamoto T, Yone K, Sakou T, Nakanishi K. Strain on intervertebral disks after anterior cervical decompression and fusion. Spine 1999;24:670–675
19. Nachemson A. The load on lumbar disks in different positions of the body. Clin Orthop 1966;45:107–122
20. Yoganandan N, Kumaresan S, Pintar FA. Biomechanics of the cervical spine, II: Cervical spine soft tissue responses and biomechanical modeling. Clin Biomech (Bristol, Avon) 2001;16:1–27
21. Panjabi MM, White AA III, Keller D, Southwick WO, Friedlaender G. Stability of the cervical spine under tension. J Biomech 1978;11:189–197
22. Dvorak J, Schneider E, Saldinger P, Rahn B. Biomechanics of the craniocervical region: the alar and transverse ligaments. J Orthop Res 1988;6:452–461
23. Hack GD, Koritzer RT, Robinson WL, Hallgren RC, Greenman PE. Anatomic relation between the rectus capitis posterior minor muscle and the dura mater. Spine 1995;20:2484–2486

24. Werne S. Studies in spontaneous atlas dislocation. Acta Orthop Scand 1957;(Suppl 23):1–150

25. Sun PP, Poffenbarger GJ, Durham S, Zimmerman RA. Spectrum of occipitoatlantoaxial injury in young children. J Neurosurg 2000;93:28–39

26. Tubbs RS, Grabb P, Spooner A, Wilson W, Oakes WJ. The apical ligament: anatomy and functional significance. J Neurosurg 2000;92:197–200

27. Goel VK, Clark CR, Gallaes K, Liu YK. Moment-rotation relationships of the ligamentous occipito-atlanto-axial complex. J Biomech 1988;21:673–680

28. Choi H. Quantitative assessment of co-contraction in cervical musculature. Med Eng Phys 2003;25:133–140

29. Patwardhan AG, Havey RM, Ghanayem AJ, et al. Load-carrying capacity of the human cervical spine in compression is increased under a follower load. Spine 2000;25:1548–1554

30. Oktenoglu T, Ozer AF, Ferrara LA, Andalkar N, Sarioglu AC, Benzel EC. Effects of cervical spine posture on axial load bearing ability: a biomechanical study. J Neurosurg 2001;94:108–114

31. Panjabi MM, White AA III, Johnson RM. Cervical spine mechanics as a function of transection of components. J Biomech 1975;8:327–336

32. White AA III, Johnson RM, Panjabi MM, Southwick WO. Biomechanical analysis of clinical stability in the cervical spine. Clin Orthop 1975;109:85–96

33. Richter M, Wilke HJ, Kluger P, Claes L, Puhl W. Load-displacement properties of the normal and injured lower cervical spine in vitro. Eur Spine J 2000;9: 104–108

34. Englander O. Nontraumatic occipito-atlanto-axial dislocation: a contribution to the radiology of the atlas. Br J Radiol 1942;15:341–345

35. Lebwohl NH, Eismont FJ. Cervical spine injuries in children. In: Weinstein SL, ed. The Pediatric Spine. New York: Raven; 1994:725–742

36. Hadley MN, Zabramski JM, Browner CM, Rekate H, Sonntag VK. Pediatric spinal trauma: review of 122 cases of spinal cord and vertebral column injuries. J Neurosurg 1988;68:18–24

37. Hamilton MG, Myles ST. Pediatric spinal injury: review of 61 deaths. J Neurosurg 1992;77:705–708

38. McGrory BJ, Klassen RA, Chao EY, Staeheli JW, Weaver AL. Acute fractures and dislocations of the cervical spine in children and adolescents. J Bone Joint Surg Am 1993;75:988–995

39. Fesmire FM, Luten RC. The pediatric cervical spine: developmental anatomy and clinical aspects. J Emerg Med 1989;7:133–142

40. Kalfas I, Wilberger J, Goldberg A, Prostko ER. Magnetic resonance imaging in acute spinal cord trauma. Neurosurgery 1988;23:295–299

41. Pang D, Wilberger JE Jr. Spinal cord injury without radiographic abnormalities in children. J Neurosurg 1982;57:114–129

42. Osenbach RK, Menezes AH. Spinal cord injury without radiographic abnormality in children. Pediatr Neurosci 1989;15:168–175

43. Ahmann PA, Smith SA, Schwartz JF, Clark DB. Spinal cord infarction due to minor trauma in children. Neurology 1975;25:301–307

44. Walsh JW, Stevens DB, Young AB. Traumatic paraplegia in children without contiguous spinal fracture or dislocation. Neurosurgery 1983;12:439–445

45. Pang D, Sahrakar K, Sun PP. Pediatric spinal cord and vertebral column injuries. In: Youmans JR, ed. Neurological Surgery: A Comprehensive Reference Guide to the Diagnosis and Management of Neurosurgical Problems. Vol 3. Philadelphia: WB Saunders; 1996:1991–2036

46. Alexander E Jr, Davis CH Jr, Field CH. Hyperextension injuries of the cervical spine. AMA Arch Neurol Psychiatry 1958;79:146–150

47. Taylor AR, Blackwood W. Paraplegia in hyperextension cervical injuries with normal radiographic appearances. J Bone Joint Surg Br 1948;30:245–248

48. Marar BC. Hyperextension injuries of the cervical spine: the pathogenesis of damage to the spinal cord. J Bone Joint Surg Am 1974;56:1655–1662

49. Burke DC. Spinal cord trauma in children. Paraplegia 1971;9:1–14

50. Glasauer FE, Cares HL. Biomechanical features of traumatic paraplegia in infancy. J Trauma 1973;13:166–170

51. Leventhal HR. Birth injuries of the spinal cord. J Pediatr 1960;56:447–453

52. Abroms IF, Bresnan MJ, Zuckerman JE, Fischer EG, Strand R. Cervical cord injuries secondary to hyperextension of the head in breech presentations. Obstet Gynecol 1973;41:369–378

53. Dickman CA, Mamourian A, Sonntag VK, Drayer BP. Magnetic resonance imaging of the transverse atlantal ligament for the evaluation of atlantoaxial instability. J Neurosurg 1991;75:221–227

54. Locke GR, Gardner JI, Van Epps EF. Atlas-dens interval (ADI) in children: a survey based on 200 normal cervical spines. Am J Roentgenol Radium Ther Nucl Med 1966;97:135–140

55. Nitecki S, Moir CR. Predictive factors of the outcome of traumatic cervical spine fracture in children. J Pediatr Surg 1994;29:1409–1411

56. Fielding JW, Cochran GB, Lawsing JF III, Hohl M. Tears of the transverse ligament of the atlas: a clinical and biomechanical study. J Bone Joint Surg Am 1974;56:1683–1691

57. Spence KF Jr, Decker S, Sell KW. Bursting atlantal fracture associated with rupture of the transverse ligament. J Bone Joint Surg Am 1970;52:543–549

58. Wholey MH, Bruwer AJ, Baker HL Jr. The lateral roentgenogram of the neck: with comments on the atlanto-odontoid-basion relationship. Radiology 1958;71:350–356

59. Bulas DI, Fitz CR, Johnson DL. Traumatic atlanto-occipital dislocation in children. Radiology 1993;188:155–158

60. Wiesel SW, Rothman RH. Occipitoatlantal hypermobility. Spine 1979;4:187–191

61. Kaufman RA, Carroll CD, Buncher CR. Atlantooccipital junction: standards for measurement in normal children. AJNR Am J Neuroradiol 1987;8:995–999

62. Harris MB, Duval MJ, Davis JA Jr, Bernini PM. Anatomical and roentgenographic features of atlantooccipital instability. J Spinal Disord 1993;6:5–10

63. Powers B, Miller MD, Kramer RS, Martinez S, Gehweiler JA Jr. Traumatic anterior atlanto-occipital dislocation. Neurosurgery 1979;4:12–17

64. Lee C, Woodring JH, Goldstein SJ, Daniel TL, Young AB, Tibbs PA. Evaluation of traumatic atlantooccipital dislocations. AJNR Am J Neuroradiol 1987;8:19–26

65. Vishteh AG, Crawford NR, Melton MS, Spetzler RF, Sonntag VK, Dickman CA. Stability of the craniovertebral junction after unilateral occipital condyle resection: a biomechanical study. J Neurosurg 1999;90:91–98

66. Pizzutillo PD, Rocha EF, D'Astous J, Kling TF Jr, McCarthy RE. Bilateral fracture of the pedicle of the second cervical vertebra in the young child. J Bone Joint Surg Am 1986;68:892–896

67. Allen B, Ferguson R. Cervical spine trauma in children. In: Bradford D, Hensinger R, eds. The Pediatric Spine. New York: Thieme; 1985

68. Roaf R. A study of the mechanics of spinal injuries. J Bone Joint Surg Br 1960;42B:810–823

69. Cusick JF, Yoganandan N. Biomechanics of the cervical spine, IV: major injuries. Clin Biomech (Bristol, Avon) 2002;17:1–20

70. White AA III, Panjabi MM. The clinical biomechanics of the occipitoatlantoaxial complex. Orthop Clin North Am 1978;9:867–878

71. White AA III, Panjabi MM. The basic kinematics of the human spine: a review of past and current knowledge. Spine 1978;3:12–20

72. Pang D, Sun PP. Pediatric vertebral column and spinal cord injuries. In: Youmans JR, ed. Neurological Surgery. Philadelphia: WB Saunders; 2004:3515–3557

# 3

# Common Pathological Conditions of the Pediatric Craniovertebral Junction and Cervical Spine

**Douglas L. Brockmeyer**

## ◆ Down Syndrome

### Etiology

Trisomy 13 is the recognized cause of Down syndrome.

### Natural History

- ◆ *Atlanto-occipital motion* There are no data examining the natural history of atlanto-occipital motion in Down syndrome patients. Fusion is recommended for atlanto-occipital motion greater than 10 mm.[1]
- ◆ *Atlantoaxial motion* The amount of C1–C2 motion remains constant over time in patients with Down syndrome once they reach ~6 years of age.[2–4] There are no data examining the natural history of atlantoaxial motion before that age. Fusion is recommended for excessive C1–C2 motion, as evidenced by an atlantodental interval greater than 6 to 8 mm or a neural canal width less than 12 mm.[1]
- ◆ *Subaxial motion* Idiopathic subaxial instability in Down syndrome is rare.[5] There are no data examining its natural history.

### Common Anatomical Idiosyncrasies

The atlanto-occipital joint in Down syndrome is characterized by a "rocker-bottom" configuration, with flat, wide occipital condyles and flat C1 articular surfaces (**Fig. 3–1**). This anatomy contributes greatly to atlanto-occipital instability. The atlas has many anatomical variants in

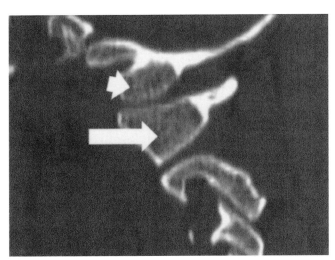

**Figure 3–1**    Parasagittal two-dimensional computed tomographic reconstruction of the occipital condyle in a typical patient with Down syndrome. It is thought that the anatomical configuration of this type of joint leads to congenital occiput–C1 instability. (arrowhead) Occipital condyle; (arrow) C1 lateral mass.

Down syndrome, although an absent or split posterior arch or a bifid arch (leading to two hemi-rings) are the two most common (**Fig. 3–2**). The axis may have odontoid abnormalities such as os odontoideum or a hypoplastic dens (**Fig. 3–3**).

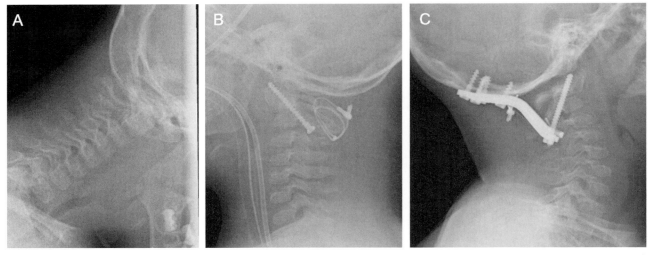

**Figure 3–2    (A)** A 3½-year-old boy with Down syndrome and atlantoaxial instability. Note congenital absence of posterior C1 ring. **(B)** Postoperative lateral cervical spine film after first fusion attempt showing C1–C2 transarticular screws and posterior bone-and-cable fusion.

**(C)** Postoperative lateral cervical spine x-ray showing second attempt at fusion with occipital–C2 construct, using C1–C2 transarticular screws and Avery-Brockmeyer-Thiokal plate (Medtronic Sofamor Danek, Minneapolis, MN).

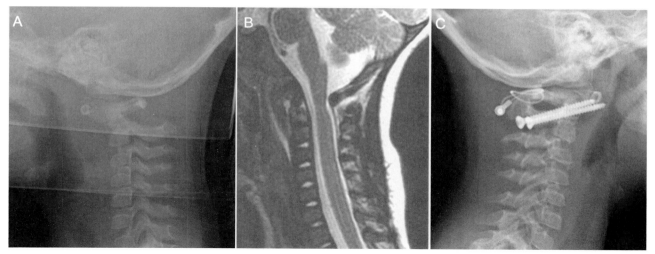

**Figure 3–3**    An 18-month-old girl with Down syndrome and severe atlantoaxial instability secondary to congenital atlantoaxial instability. **(A)** Preoperative lateral plain film, showing severe atlantoaxial instability. **(B)** Preoperative midsagittal T2-weighted magnetic resonance imaging, showing narrowing at the craniovertebral junction. **(C)** Postoperative lateral plain x-ray, showing C1–C2 transarticular screws and posterior bone-and-cable "girth-hitch" arthrodesis.

## Surgical Considerations

Posterior C1–C2 transarticular screw fixation is an excellent method to provide internal stability for Down syndrome patients at almost any age. However, care must be taken in patients with posterior C1 arch abnormalities because there may not be enough bone available to provide an environment for adequate fusion. For patients with atlanto-occipital instability, an occiput to C2 fusion with internal fixation, such as the Avery-Brockmeyer-Thiokol (ABT) plate (Medtronic Sofamor Danek, Minneapolis, MN ), is a very good construct.

## ◆ Klippel-Feil Syndrome and Klippel-Feil Variant

### Etiology

The etiology of Klippel-Feil syndrome and Klippel-Feil variant is unknown. Multiple theories have been proposed, but a vascular etiology seems most likely.[6,7]

### Natural History

Instability caused by intrinsic abnormalities of the craniocervical joints may progress over time. One study found cervicothoracic fusions to be a risk

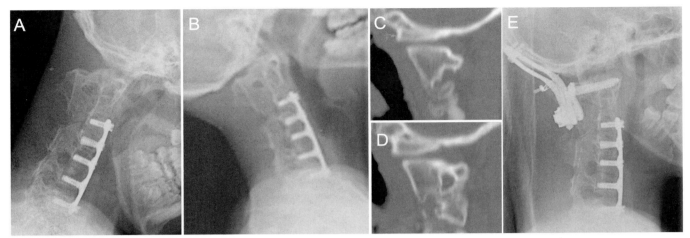

**Figure 3–4** A 10-year-old girl with Klippel-Feil syndrome, with a history of previous anterior cervical diskectomy and fusion from C3 to C7. **(A)** Plain lateral cervical spine film in flexion, showing significant incursion of the occiput on C2. **(B)** Plain lateral cervical spine film in extension, showing reduction of deformity from the previous figure. **(C,D)** Parasagittal two-dimensional computed tomographic reconstructions through the occipital condyle of the **(C)** right and **(D)** left C1–C2 regions, respectively. Note the extremely flat shape of the occipital condyle/C1 region. **(E)** Postoperative plain lateral cervical spine film, showing occiput–upper cervical spine fusion using Ohio Medical Instruments (OMI) loop (Ohio Medical Instruments Company, Inc., Cincinnati, OH) and C1 lateral mass screws bilaterally.

factor for progressive instability.[8] Adjacent level instability may occur after fusion of any craniocervical segment (**Fig. 3–4**).

### Common Anatomical Idiosyncrasies

Klippel-Feil syndrome and its variants are commonly associated with occipitalization of the atlas, Chiari I malformation, and a wide variety of complex, sometimes bizarre, cervical bony abnormalities (**Figs. 3–5, 3–6,** and **3–7**). Bone quality is typically normal.

### Surgical Considerations

As a group, Klippel-Feil syndrome patients present with a wide variety of craniocervical pathologies, leading to use of the entire spectrum of craniocervical surgical techniques. Great care must be taken in the preoperative phase to understand the patient's anatomy so that surgical planning takes into account all possible ways of achieving stability. The surgeon will be significantly challenged in a high percentage of cases.

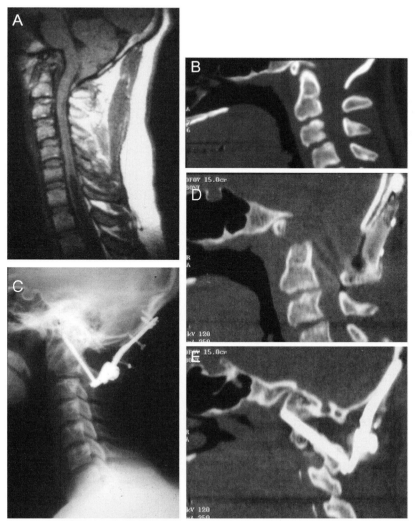

**Figure 3–5**    A 15-year-old boy with occipitalization of the atlas, Chiari 1 malformation, and severe ventral brain stem compression. Physical examination showed bulbar and myelopathic findings. **(A)** Lateral midsagittal T1-weighted magnetic resonance imaging showing severe ventral brain stem compression and Chiari 1 malformation.
**(B)** Preoperative midsagittal two-dimensional computed tomographic (CT) reconstruction of the craniovertebral junction showing occipitalization of the atlas.
**(C)** Postoperative plain lateral cervical spine film, showing occipital–C2 fusion, using preformed loop (Ohio Medical Instruments Company, Inc., Cincinnati, OH) and bone-and-cable arthrodesis. **(D)** Late postoperative midsagittal two-dimensional CT reconstruction of the craniovertebral junction, showing solid bony arthrodesis from the occiput–C2 and the removal of the odontoid tip ventrally. **(E)** Postoperative parasagittal two-dimensional CT reconstruction, showing path of C1–C2 transarticular screw coupled with Ohio Medical Instruments (OMI) loop.

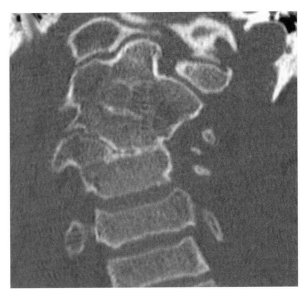

**Figure 3–6**   Coronal two-dimensional computed tomographic reconstruction of the craniovertebral area in a patient with Klippel-Feil and severe congenital bony anomalies and scoliotic angulation between C2 and C3.

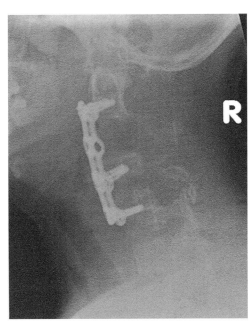

**Figure 3–7**   Plain lateral cervical spine film, taken postoperatively from a 14-year-old girl with Klippel-Feil syndrome and severe multilevel cervical instability. This anterior ABC plate (Aesculap, Inc., Center Valley, PA) was coupled with a posterior bone-and-cable fusion to provide solid bony arthrodesis.

## ◆ Neurofibromatosis Type 1

### Etiology

Mutation in the neurofibromatosis type 1 (NF1) gene located on chromosome 17q causes neurofibromatosis type 1.

### Natural History

Progressive cervical kyphosis may occur because of intrinsic ligamentous abnormality and abnormal bony architecture (**Fig. 3–8**). Cervical kyphosis may also occur following resection of soft tissue or extradural neurofibromas. No studies have examined this topic in children.

### Common Anatomical Idiosyncrasies

Scalloping of the vertebral column is common but does not necessarily cause cervical instability. Bone quality is typically poorer than average, and rigid internal fixation is important.

### Surgical Considerations

Reconstruction of the cervical spine for kyphotic abnormalities is typically performed first from the anterior direction with multilevel diskectomies, fusions, and plating at the appropriate level, followed by posterior rib

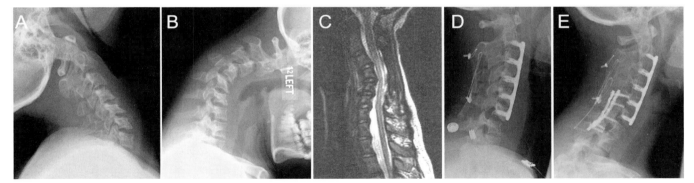

**Figure 3–8**  A 14-year-old girl with neurofibromatosis and idiopathic swan-neck deformity. **(A)** Preoperative plain x-ray in extension. **(B)** Preoperative plain x-ray in flexion showing severe kyphotic angulation centered at approximately C4–C5. **(C)** Preoperative magnetic resonance imaging demonstrating multilevel canal narrowing. **(D)** Postoperative plain films showing anterior plate and screw construct between C2 and C6, with posterior bone-and-cable fusion from C2 to C6. Note bilateral jumped facets at C6–C7. **(E)** Follow-up plain lateral radiograph taken 1 year following surgery, showing extension of fused levels from C5 to T1 in the posterior direction augmented by posterior bone and cable fusion. The ABC system (Aesculap, Inc., Center Valley, PA) was used in the anterior direction, and small-notched plates (Synthes, Inc., West Chester, PA) were used from the posterior direction.

and cable arthrodesis if necessary. Achieving normal cervical alignment is the goal.

## ◆ Os Odontoideum

### Etiology

The exact etiology of os odontoideum is unknown. Congenital and posttraumatic origins have been proposed, with a posttraumatic origin likely in most cases.[9,10]

### Natural History

The natural history of os odontoideum is variable, and predictive factors for deterioration, particularly in the asymptomatic patient, have not been identified. The literature provides many examples of both asymptomatic and symptomatic patients with known os odontoideum who had not undergone surgery and who had not reported problems in follow-up over many years.[11] Conversely, examples of sudden spinal cord injury in association with os odontoideum following minor trauma have also been reported.[12] Given the fact that the dens, a major stabilizing structure of the atlantoaxial joint, is incompetent in an os odontoideum, operative fusion is usually indicated.

### Common Anatomical Idiosyncrasies

The literature describes two types of os odontoideum: orthotopic and dystopic. A dystopic os odontoideum is functionally connected to the basion, whereas an orthotopic os odontoideum moves with the anterior arch of the atlas. Orthotopic os odontoideum is much more common than the dystopic variety. Atlantoaxial rotatory subluxation may also occur as part of the instability and must be reduced prior to internal fixation.

### Surgical Considerations

An os odontoideum may be regarded as the prototypical indication for posterior C1–C2 transarticular screw fixation with bone and cable fusion (**Figs. 3–9, 3–10,** and **3–11**). Careful preoperative planning is necessary to place the transarticular screws safely. A patient with a highly unstable os odontoideum with cord compression should be turned from the supine to the prone position in the operating room with a hard collar in place to protect against further spinal cord injury. A subluxed os odontoideum may be reduced intraoperatively by manipulating C2 either dorsally or ventrally just prior to passing the drill bit through the C1–C2 interspace into the lateral mass of C1.

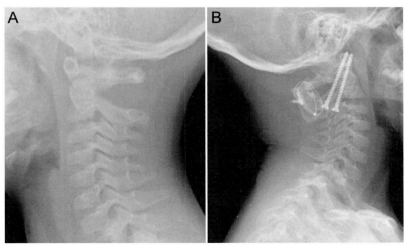

**Figure 3–9**   A 6-year-old boy with os odontoideum. **(A)** Plain lateral cervical spine film showing the presence of os odontoideum. **(B)** Postoperative plain lateral cervical spine film showing solid arthrodesis between C1 and C2, along with C1–C2 transarticular screws.

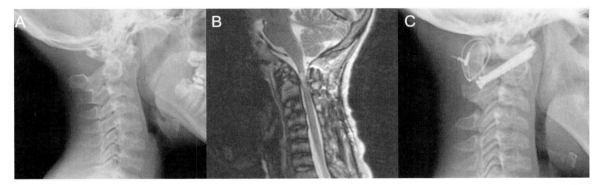

**Figure 3–10**   A 10-year-old boy with spinal epiphyseal dysplasia, os odontoideum, and severe canal narrowing. **(A)** Plain lateral cervical spine film in neutral position. **(B)** Midsagittal T2-weighted magnetic resonance imaging showing severe canal narrowing and high signal intensity suggestive of cord injury. **(C)** Postoperative lateral cervical spine film showing placement of C1–C2 transarticular screws and solid bony arthrodesis at the posterior C1–C2 level.

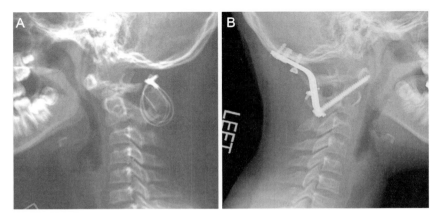

**Figure 3–11**   A 14-year-old boy with os odontoideum and a history of two previous failed fusion attempts between C1 and C2, with bone-and-wire arthrodesis. **(A)** Plain lateral cervical spine film showing bone-and-cable arthrodesis with fusion failure and pulling out of the wires, along with the posterior arch of C1. **(B)** Postoperative lateral cervical spine film showing occiput–C2 fusion construct, using C1–C2 transarticular screws, ABT plate (Medtronic Sofamor Danek, Memphis, TN), and occiput–C2 bone-and-cable fusion.

## ◆ Common Skeletal Dysplasias

### Etiology

1. *Morquio's syndrome* Morquio's syndrome, or mucopolysaccharidosis IV, is an autosomal recessive disorder. Type A (severe) and type B (mild) are recognized by the enzymes involved.
2. *Spondyloepiphyseal dysplasia* Spondyloepiphyseal dysplasia (SED) is an autosomal dominant disorder.
3. *Diastrophic dwarfism* Diastrophic dwarfism is an autosomal recessive disorder.

### Natural History

These skeletal dysplasias are characterized by diminished stature and shortened life span. Bone quality may be below average but is usually adequate to obtain successful fusion. The patient may or may not have normal mentation.

### Common Anatomical Idiosyncrasies

A hypoplastic or aplastic dens is common in these syndromes, with varying degrees of atlantoaxial subluxation present. Os odontoideum is relatively rare.

### Surgical Considerations

Size-for-age considerations are a major challenge. For example, a 10-year-old patient with SED may be the size of a normal 4-year-old (**Fig. 3–12**). The

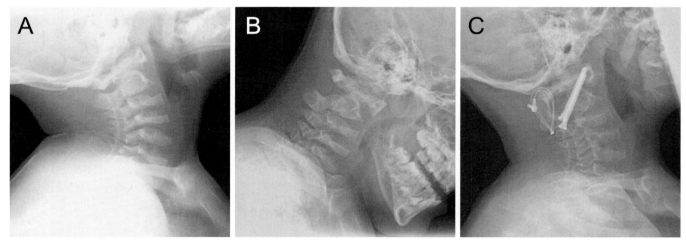

**Figure 3–12**    A 10-year-old boy with metatrophic dwarfism, hypoplastic odontoid, and atlantoaxial instability. **(A)** Preoperative lateral x-ray in extension. **(B)** Preoperative lateral x-ray in flexion, with severe atlantoaxial instability. **(C)** Postoperative lateral plain x-ray with C1–C2 transarticular screws and posterior bone-and-cable fusion.

surgical challenge of placing adequate instrumentation, especially C1–C2 transarticular screws, may be extreme (**Figs. 3–13** and **3–14**). With proper preoperative planning and careful attention to detail during surgery, however, these patients can undergo rigid screw fixation and go on to successful fusion without the use of an external halo orthosis.

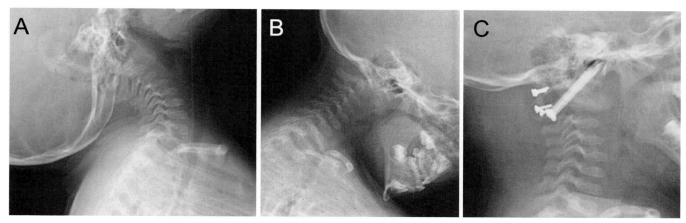

**Figure 3–13**   A 5-year-old girl with spondyloepiphyseal dysplasia and atlantoaxial instability with congenital absence of the posterior arch of C1 and hypoplastic odontoid. **(A)** Preoperative lateral plain x-ray in extension. **(B)** Preoperative lateral plain x-ray in flexion showing severe atlantoaxial instability. Note absence of posterior C1 elements. **(C)** Postoperative lateral plain film, showing C1–C2 transarticular screws with rib-and-screw fixation between the posterior elements of C2 and the posterolateral elements of the C1 arch.

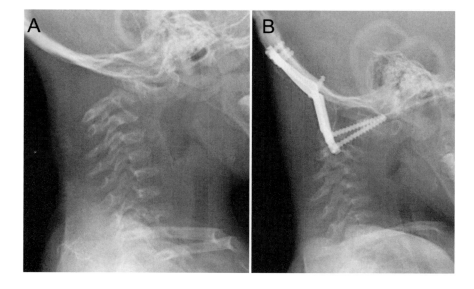

**Figure 3–14**   A 3-year-old boy with undetermined skeletal dysplasia and severe craniovertebral kyphosis. **(A)** Preoperative lateral plain x-ray in neutral position. **(B)** Preoperative lateral plain x-ray, showing occipital–C2 fusion with C1–C2 transarticular screws and bone–cable–screw arthrodesis from occiput to C2.

## References

### Down Syndrome

1. Brockmeyer D. Down syndrome and craniovertebral instability: topic review and treatment recommendations. Pediatr Neurosurg 1999;31:71–77
2. Morton R, Khan M, Murray-Leslie C, Elliot S. Atlantoaxial instability in Down's syndrome: a five-year follow-up study. Arch Dis Child 1995;72:115–119
3. Pueschel S, Scola F, Pezzullo J. A longitudinal study of atlanto-dens relationships in asymptomatic individuals with Down syndrome. Pediatrics 1992;89: 1194–1198
4. Ferguson R, Putney M, Allen B. Comparison of neurologic deficits with atlanto-dens intervals in patients with Down syndrome. J Spinal Disord 1997;10:246–252
5. Citow JS, Munshi I, Chang-Stroman T, Sullivan C, Frim DM. C2/3 instability in a child with Down's syndrome: case report and discussion. Pediatr Neurosurg 1998;28:143–146

### Klippel-Feil Syndrome and Klippel-Feil Variant

6. Brill CB, Peyster RG, Keller MS, Galtman L. Isolation of the right subclavian artery with subclavian steal in a child with Klippel-Feil anomaly: an example of the subclavian artery supply disruption sequence. Am J Med Genet 1987;26:933–940
7. Bavinck JN, Weaver DD. Subclavian artery supply disruption sequence: hypothesis of a vascular etiology for Poland, Klippel-Feil, and Mobius anomalies. Am J Med Genet 1986;23:903–918
8. Pizzutillo P, Woods M, Nicholson L, MacEwen G. Risk factors in Klippel-Feil syndrome. Spine 1994;19:2110–2116

### Os Odontoideum

9. Verska J, Anderson P. Os odontoideum: a case report of one identical twin. Spine 1997;22:706–709
10. Morgan M, Onofrio B, Bender C. Familial os odontoideum: case report. J Neurosurg 1989;70:636–639
11. Spierings E, Braakman R. The management of os odontoideum: analysis of 37 cases. J Bone Joint Surg Br 1982;64:422–428
12. Menezes AH, Ryken TC. Craniovertebral abnormalities in Down's syndrome. Pediatr Neurosurg 1992;18:24–33

# 4

# Traumatic Injuries of the Pediatric Craniocervical Junction

**Marcus L. Ware, Kurtis I. Auguste, Nalin Gupta, Peter P. Sun, and Douglas L. Brockmeyer**

Traumatic injuries of the pediatric craniocervical complex occur at a high frequency. Therefore, we dedicate a separate chapter to considering the various injuries that can occur. Each injury or injury pattern is discussed in detail, starting with its definition, clinical presentation, radiographic diagnosis, and treatment, so that pediatric spine surgeons may better understand the nature of these injuries.

As discussed in earlier chapters, injury to the pediatric spine differs from injury to the adult spine in several important ways. These include the anatomical and biomechanical features of the pediatric spine, the mechanism of injury, injury pattern, criteria for determining instability, and outcome. The pediatric craniocervical complex is particularly susceptible to injury. There are four major injury patterns in the pediatric craniocervical junction: (1) longitudinal subluxation with failure of the major stabilizers across the occiput–C2 (O–C2) unit, (2) translational atlantoaxial subluxation, (3) atlantoaxial rotatory fixation, and (4) fractures. There are also four major injury patterns in the pediatric subaxial spine: (1) ligamentous and soft tissue disruption, (2) bony anterior column injuries, (3) bony posterior column injures, and (4) combined anterior and posterior column, injuries. Each injury pattern is discussed in turn, with relevant details provided for the management of complex injuries in the craniocervical complex in children.

## ◆ Craniovertebral Junction Injuries

### Longitudinal Occiput–C2 Subluxation

*Injury Description* Longitudinal subluxation results in the separation of the occiput to C1 or C1 to C2 or both. The former pattern is more common, and the injury is commonly referred to as atlanto-occipital (A-O) dislocation. Autopsy studies of children with fatal atlanto-occipital dislocations often reveal disruption of all ligaments connecting the occiput to the atlas and axis as well as transection of the spinal cord or brain stem.[1–3] Rupture of either or both the tectorial membrane and alar ligaments invariably occurs with rupture of the joint capsule. The posterior cervical and suboccipital musculature is sprained or lacerated, and the prevertebral fascia is infiltrated with blood. There are usually no fractures. In older children and adults, stronger ligaments can result in avulsion fractions at the ligamentous attachment of the occipital condyle or the base of the clivus as opposed to rupture of the ligaments themselves.[3–5]

The exact vectors of impact that create this injury are not known. The incidence of associated facial injuries, particularly submental lacerations and mandibular fractures, is high.[3] Posterior atlas fractures with posterior atlanto-occipital dislocations have also been observed in adults.[6] These findings are consistent with a hyperextension injury. Furthermore, nine of 12 victims of atlanto-occipital dislocation in Adams's autopsy study sustained pontomedullary lacerations,[3] which are associated with hyperextension[7,8] and rotational injuries.[9] Approximately 25% of reported atlanto-occipital dislocations, however, have coexistent atlantoaxial subluxation or separation of the posterior elements of atlas and axis, suggesting a hyperflexion injury.[10] Autopsy studies also reveal spinomedullary contusions or transections adjacent to the dens where the tectorial membrane is disrupted, as if the dens protrudes through the tectorial membrane during extreme flexion.[3,11] Lateral flexion and extreme rotation are also thought to play a role in this injury type.[12–14] Taken together, these reports suggest that atlanto-occipital dislocation can probably occur as a result of either hyperflexion or hyperextension that tears the tectorial membrane, in combination with extreme rotation, lateral flexion, and distraction that disrupts the alar ligaments.

***Clinical Presentation***  In the past, atlanto-occipital dislocation was considered a rare and usually fatal injury.[15] More recently, a larger number of survivors, especially children, have been reported.[14–19] Several factors may contribute to the increase in survival, including quicker response times to the scene by emergency medical teams, better initial cervical spine immobilization, and earlier diagnosis of injury.

Children with traumatic atlanto-occipital dislocation usually present with cardiorespiratory instability and neurological findings indicating brain stem, spinal cord, and cranial nerve injuries. In several studies, 30% of children who survived atlanto-occipital dislocation were apneic or in full cardiorespiratory arrest at the accident scene.[15,16,19–24] Neurological findings indicating brain stem injury include pupillary abnormalities, rotatory nystagmus, ocular bobbing, and decerebrate posturing. Motor deficits vary depending on the level and degree of injury. The caudal six pairs of cranial nerves are frequently injured. Axial traction of the medulla may stretch or avulse the lower cranial nerves from their exit foramen at the base of the skull.[25] Subsequent difficulty with aspiration and swallowing confers significant morbidity. Positive computed tomographic (CT) scans of the head in children with atlanto-occipital dislocation most commonly show diffuse swelling, with subarachnoid blood in the basal cisterns or intraventricular blood in the III and IV ventricles. Acute and delayed hydrocephalus with syringomyelia have been observed.[21,26]

Because complete cervicomedullary disruption is fatal, most survivors of atlanto-occipital dislocation have incomplete injuries and will improve. Cranial nerve palsies, however, tend to persist. Children who survive the initial crisis may make good recovery despite their having severe presenting neurological deficits.

***Radiographic Diagnosis*** The diagnosis of atlanto-occipital dislocation requires diligent analysis. This injury may be suspected in high-speed trauma victims, especially those with facial injuries and cardiorespiratory instability. Longitudinal O–C2 dislocation on plain radiographs of survivors may be subtle and is frequently missed. Early diagnosis is crucial to prevent additional devastating neurological injury. The first clue is often widening of the retropharyngeal space beyond 7 mm seen on lateral cervical radiographs. Several criteria based on the relationship of key anatomical landmarks have been proposed to recognize O–C2 instability; these are outlined in the discussion of craniovertebral biomechanics in Chapter 2.

All patients with suspicious findings on plain radiographs, based on any of the described criteria, should undergo  CT and magnetic resonance imaging (MRI) from the occiput to C2 with reconstructed sagittal and coronal images. In cases of atlanto-occipital dislocation, a sagittal CT reconstruction through the atlanto-occipital joint often demonstrates an abnormal separation or translation of the cup-shaped articulation. In subtle cases of longitudinal separation, the adjacent joint diastasis serves as a comparison. MRI can delineate the disruption of the ligaments with a complete tear or bowing of the tectorial membrane (**Fig. 4–1**). Furthermore, the extent of brain stem and spinal cord damage and the presence of associated structural compression can be seen

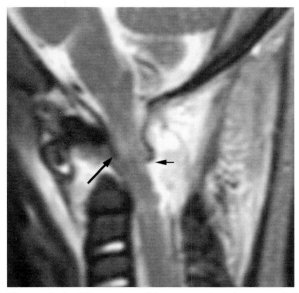

**Figure 4–1**   Disruption of ligaments in atlanto-occipital dislocation. The long arrow shows magnetic resonance imaging evidence of a tear in the tectorial membrane. The short arrow shows evidence of blood layering posterior to the dura.

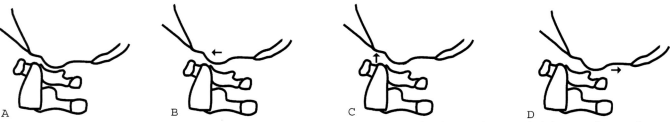

**Figure 4–2**   Traynelis classification of atlanto-occipital dislocation. **(A)** Normal; **(B)** type I (anterior); **(C)** type II (vertical); **(D)** type III (posterior).

with MRI. In cases where atlanto-occipital dislocation is reduced at presentation, plain films and CT may fail to demonstrate any bony abnormality. These injuries have been reported to become apparent only with traction, a precarious situation.[27]

Traynelis and colleagues have classified atlanto-occipital dislocation into three types (**Fig. 4–2**).[10] Type I is characterized by the anterior displacement of the occiput relative to the atlas; type II is characterized by a longitudinal separation between the two structures; and type III is associated with the posterior displacement of the occiput. In addition to these three types, isolated examples of pure lateral dislocation as well as pure rotatory subluxation have been reported in children, the latter with atlantoaxial rotatory fixation.[28–30] The majority of traumatic atlanto-occipital dislocations in children are type I. Given the highly unstable nature of this injury in children, the direction of occipital displacement may be more a function of patient positioning than of the mechanism of injury. As a child lies on a flat board, the larger head relative to the thorax will flex the neck. If atlanto-occipital dislocation exists, the displacement will tend to be anterior. In 1948, Farthing reported the only case of traumatic type III dislocation seen in a child where the child's neck was extended on presentation.[31] Because axial stabilization of the entire O–C2 unit is supplied by the ligaments from the occiput to C2, longitudinal abnormalities at the C1–C2 articulation can be considered a different manifestation of the same injury.[32] Anderson and Montesano propose that this injury is a variant of type II atlanto-occipital dislocation (type IIb).[33]

***Treatment***   Management of atlanto-occipital dislocation begins with rapid cardiorespiratory resuscitation. Immobilization must be provided immediately and maintained until definitive stabilization. The use of cervical traction or failure to provide immobilization can have catastrophic consequences. Immobilization should be provided with a cervical collar until halo orthosis can be applied. Neutral positioning alone during initial immobilization in a cervical collar can help reduce atlanto-occipital dislocations without the need for traction. As mentioned, the larger head of the child relative to the torso tends to flex the neck and maintain an anterior dislocation. Elevation of the thorax with firm padding or blankets with the child placed in the cervical collar can eliminate the size discrepancy and help reduce the dislocation. An oversized collar can exacerbate longitudinal distraction, even with the child in a neutral position. The reverse Trendelenburg position with elevation of the head in a proper collar can correct a type II dislocation.

Definitive stabilization requires surgical fusion. Although spontaneous fibrous fusion with immobilization alone has been reported in children,[12,26,34] persistent instability is generally the rule because purely ligamentous spinal injuries heal poorly.[14,16,31,35] In such cases, fusion across the entire O–C2 unit must be strongly considered. Although overt C1–C2 separation from disruption of the O–C2 connections may be visualized, covert C1–C2 instability cannot be separately elicited in the presence of O–C1 separation. In fact, C1–C2 longitudinal instability may be assumed, given the failure of the ligaments from the occiput to C2.

## Atlantoaxial Rotatory Subluxation

***Injury Description***   Atlantoaxial rotatory subluxation (AARS) consists of a spectrum of rotational abnormalities involving the atlas and the axis, including atlantoaxial rotatory fixation (AARF). This spectrum ranges from mild abnormalities of rotation to absolute fixation with no motion. AARS may arise from several potential mechanisms. In some cases, physiological hypermobility of the atlantoaxial articulation in children may lead to rotatory subluxation during sudden and vigorous turning of the head.[36] This can occasionally cause a true bony lock. In other cases, the redundant synovial folds in children may become trapped in joint spaces at the extreme of rotation and cause a jam during counterrotation. Concurrent muscle spasms may then exacerbate this fixation.

***Clinical Presentation***   AARS often occurs with little or no preceding trauma.[37,38] This injury has been described after infections of the head and neck, such as pharyngitis, otitis media, retropharyngeal abscesses, or tumors.[39] Torticollis after pharyngeal inflammation has been called Grisel's syndrome. Traumatic AARS occurs in only 30% of cases of AARS, and the trauma is usually minor. Children present with neck pain, with the neck maintained in lateral flexion and the chin rotated to the contralateral side (a "cock-robin deformity"). The neurological examination is usually normal, Rarely, patients present with myelopathy or C2 radiculopathy.[40,41] Since its first description in 1830,[42] several reports of this condition have been published, but the diagnostic criteria are under debate.

***Radiographic Diagnosis***   Fielding and Hawkins devised a classification scheme for AARS based on analysis of plain films.[41] In their study, four types of AARS are described. Type I rotatory subluxation is characterized by rotatory fixation without anterior shift of the atlas. This is the most common type described in children and is the most stable because the transverse ligament should remain intact. Type II consists of rotatory subluxation with an anterior shift of greater than 3 mm but less than 5 mm. This type involves compromise of the transverse ligament and is more dangerous. Type III involves rotatory subluxation with an anterior shift of greater than 5 mm. Type IV is a rare and usually fatal injury that involves rotatory fixation with a posterior shift. The relationship of C1 to C2 can be well visualized with three-dimensional CT scans (**Fig. 4–3**). Recent studies using dynamic CT have also successfully visualized AARS and AARF.[39,43] Lee and Pang have used deviation from the normal C1–C2 motion curve described in Chapter 2 to diagnose AARS.[44]

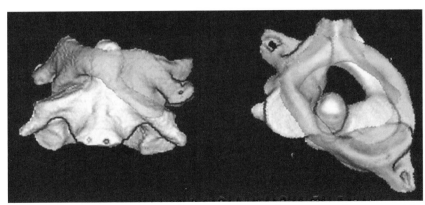

**Figure 4–3**    Three-dimensional reconstruction of a computed tomographic scan of a patient with type I atlantoaxial rotatory fixation. (Courtesy of Dr. Ronald Cohen at the Children's Hospital at Oakland.)

*Treatment*    The treatment for AARS may consist of conservative therapy alone, nonsteroidal anti-inflammatory drugs, muscle relaxants, use of a soft collar or hard cervical collar, halter traction, cervicothoracic orthosis, halo traction, and cervical fusion. The majority of patients with type I injury improve with a combination of medical therapy and traction.[39,43,45] Once reduction of the injury is achieved, immobilization for 4 to 6 weeks in a collar is recommended. Studies have shown that the duration of symptoms prior to treatment is a critical factor in determining the response to more conservative treatment.[39] Recurrences of type I injuries may indicate transverse ligament incompetence and may require C1–C2 fusion. Type II and III injuries should be considered inherently unstable because of injury to the transverse ligament and require C1–C2 fusion.

### Translational Atlantoaxial Subluxation

*Injury Description*    Translational atlantoaxial subluxation without fracture occurs when there is ligamentous instability. Loss of the transverse ligament allows the spinal cord to become compressed between the odontoid and the posterior arch of the atlas. Traumatic translational atlantoaxial subluxation is an extremely rare injury in children that occurs as the result of violent trauma, with few survivors.[46,47] Most cases of traumatic translational atlantoaxial subluxation result from flexion injuries[48]; however, there are rare injuries with posterior C1–C2 subluxation in the presence of a normal odontoid and C1 ring caused by hyperextension or C1–C2 distraction.[49] Nontraumatic translational instability of C1–C2 is associated with laxity of the transverse ligament or hypoplasia of the odontoid. This occurs in several developmental disorders, including Down syndrome, Klippel-Feil syndrome, and many of the skeletal dysplasias.

*Clinical Presentation*    In most patients who present with translational atlantoaxial subluxation, the injuries result from high-speed pedestrian–vehicular accidents.[37,50,51] Patients present at two extremes. They generally have only minor neck pain, subtle myelopathy, or C2 hypesthesia, or they have severe head injury that is often exacerbated by anoxic encephalopathy. Long-term survivors often recover with good function.

***Radiographic Diagnosis*** The diagnosis of translational atlantoaxial subluxation can often be made with a lateral cervical x-ray. In the absence of other fractures, an atlantodental interval (ADI) of greater than 4 mm is considered abnormal in children,[52–54] though some accept the normal to be up to 5 mm.[52,55] As the ADI exceeds 6 to 10 mm, the alar ligaments and tectorial membrane become secondarily damaged, and A-O instability ensues. The retropharyngeal soft tissues are usually widened. In some cases, MRI may show rupture of the transverse ligament.[56,57] Occasionally, flexion–extension films of the cervical spine are required to show instability.

***Treatment*** Although immobilization has been attempted in children with translational C1–C2 subluxation, it is generally accepted that the extensive ligamentous injury must be treated by C1–C2 fusion.[37,52,53] Postoperative halo immobilization may be avoided with transarticular screw fixation.[58]

## Odontoid Fractures

***Injury Description*** True odontoid fractures are rare in children. The odontoid synchondrosis is located between the dens and the C2 body and is normally fused by 11 years of age. In children less than 11 years of age, C1 on C2 subluxations are usually a result of epiphyseal separation, or epiphysiolysis, between the odontoid and the body of C2. Fortunately, this fracture tends to decompress the cord and is thus less likely to lead to neurological deficit. Most odontoid synchondrosis fractures occur in children under 3 years of age.[59]

***Clinical Presentation*** The majority of children with odontoid epiphysiolysis present after severe falls or after motor vehicle accidents; however, children may present after much milder trauma. Neck pain is a common complaint. Because a high percentage of cervical injuries are also associated with head trauma,[60] children may be obtunded from concurrent head injury. However, many children who present with odontoid injuries are neurologically intact because injury to the cord at this level is often fatal.

***Radiographic Diagnosis*** In cases of true odontoid fracture or epiphysiolysis, lateral radiographs usually show an anteriorly displaced odontoid process with a normal ADI. In odontoid epiphysiolysis, evaluation by CT may show a widened growth plate (**Fig. 4–4**). Anterior angulations of the odontoid fragment are often seen.

***Treatment*** There are few recommendations for treatment of odontoid injuries in children. Mandabach et al described treatment of 13 children with odontoid injuries ranging from 9 months to 7 years of age.[61] Eight of 10 children achieved stable fusion after immobilization with a halo orthosis over a range of 10 to 18 weeks. Sherk reported that only 1 of 35 children with an odontoid injury required surgical fusion.[62] Taken together, these reports suggest that early immobilization of children after injury should be sufficient in most cases. In cases of failed fusion after immobilization, C1–C2 fusion is recommended[63] (**Fig. 4–5**).

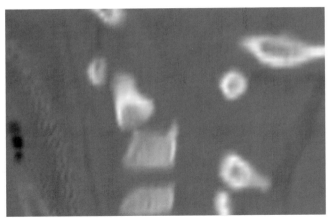

**Figure 4–4**    Midsagittal two-dimensional reconstruction and thin-cut computed tomographic scan depicting an odontoid synchondrosis fracture with anterolisthesis of the odontoid fragment ~3 mm forward from the C2 body.

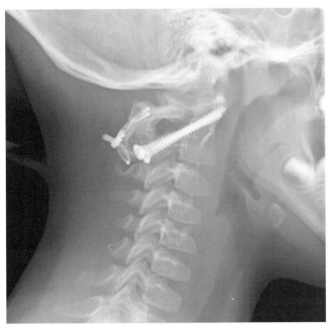

**Figure 4–5**    Postoperative plain lateral cervical spine film depicting placement of C1–C2 transarticular screws and a successful posterior atlantoaxial fusion in a 2-year-old child.

## C2 Pedicle Fractures

*Injury Description* The C2 pedicle fracture, also called hangman's fracture, is rare in the pediatric population. No data are available on the mechanism of this injury in children, although it is thought to be similar to that in adults.

*Clinical Presentation* Only a few cases of neurological deficit associated with C2 pedicle fracture injury in children have been reported. Pizzutillo et al reported a case series of five patients in which only one of the five had neurological deficit.[64] There is a single report of central cord syndrome after C2 pedicle fracture.[65]

*Radiographic Diagnosis* Diagnosis of C2 pedicle fractures can be difficult even with a high index of suspicion. The neural central synchondrosis can mimic fracture on oblique radiographs in children under the age of 7 years. In addition, pseudosubluxation at C2–C3 is present in many children and may also mimic subluxation. In such cases, evaluation by CT may be helpful.

*Treatment* Treatment of C2 fractures in children is similar to that in adults.[59] If the body of C2 is not significantly displaced on C3, immobilization in a rigid collar should be adequate. In cases of greater than 3 mm of anterior displacement, a Minerva cast or halo would be more appropriate. Surgical fusion is rarely required.

## ◆ Subaxial Cervical Spine Injuries

### Ligamentous and Soft Tissue Injury

*Injury Description* Subaxial ligamentous and soft tissue injury can be defined as any injury to the supporting structures of the bony cervical spine below C2. It can range from a very mild injury to severe disruption of all the supporting structures, leading to gross spinal instability. The ligamentous and soft tissue structures of the cervical spine include the anterior and posterior longitudinal ligaments, disk material, capsular facet ligaments, interspinous ligaments, and all the supporting muscles and muscular attachments. Taken in its entirety, it is presumed that subaxial ligamentous and soft tissue disruption, including myofascial pain syndromes, is by far the most common type of cervical spine injury in children and accounts for a significant amount of discomfort and disability.

*Clinical Presentation* Unless comatose, all patients present with neck pain. Neurological deficit, including either radiculopathy, myelopathy, or both, may be seen, depending on the severity of the injury. Neck pain that persists for several weeks after an accident is uncommon in children and should be investigated with radiological studies.

*Radiographic Diagnosis* Patients with subaxial ligamentous and soft tissue injury have a wide variety of potential radiographic abnormalities, ranging from completely normal studies to grossly abnormal findings. Static plain cervical spine films should be normal but may exhibit instability on flexion and extension if enough injury is present to destabilize the spine. Criteria for determining subaxial stability are subluxation of more than 5 mm or kyphotic angulation greater than 15 degrees. Pang (unpublished data) has shown evidence that a kyphotic angulation of greater than 7 degrees represents significant ligamentous injury and predisposes the juvenile cervical spine to further kyphosis and instability. The instability is typically at one level but may encompass two if the injury is particularly severe. CT scans should show normal bone anatomy, but sagittal reconstructions may show evidence of cervical subluxation. MRI, especially short T1 inversion recovery (STIR) images, is particularly helpful in establishing the diagnosis. High signal is seen in the soft tissues, and blood products may be seen in disrupted disk spaces or ligaments. A "reverse L" sign seen on the STIR images in the posterior interspinous tissue at one or more subaxial cervical levels is highly suspicious of a significant ligamentous and soft tissue injury to the spine (**Fig. 4–6**).

*Treatment* Subaxial ligamentous and soft tissue injury is typically managed in a conservative fashion, using oral analgesics and a cervical collar, if necessary. The patient's paravertebral muscle spasm usually resolves within 1 to 2 weeks

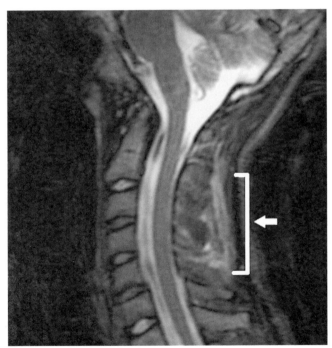

**Figure 4–6**   Midsagittal cervical spine magnetic resonance imaging with short T1 inversion recovery sequence. Arrows depict "reverse L" sign, indicative of posterior ligamentous cervical spine injury.

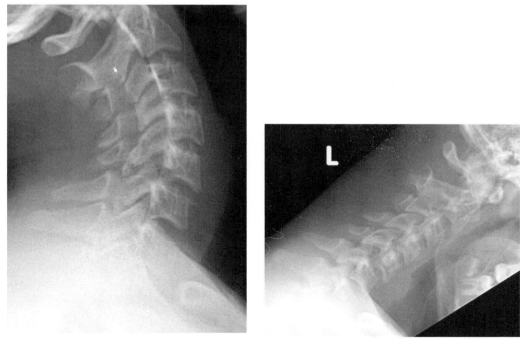

**Figure 4–7**  Preoperative lateral cervical spine film in a 14-year-old boy after trauma. **(A)** Extension film shows reduction of subluxation. **(B)** Flexion film shows anterolisthesis of C5 on C6 of ~5 mm.

after the injury, although an occasional patient might have discomfort for a month or more. Finch and Barnes[66] used primary operative stabilization in most children with ligamentous injury. However, they stated that in at least some of these cases, external immobilization may have resulted in ligamentous healing. Pennecot et al[67] treated minor ligamentous injuries with reduction and collar inmobilization; however, 8 of 11 children with subaxial ligamentous injury required fusion. Patients who have enough ligamentous or soft tissue injury to result in spinal instability must be managed surgically (**Fig. 4–7A,B**). Anterior cervical diskectomy and fusion, with either allograft (preferred) or autograft, is performed at the involved levels, followed by plate and screw fixation (**Fig. 4–8**). Posterior fusion and plating may also be performed, depending on surgeon preference. Occasionally, the instability is so severe that both anterior and posterior fusion must be performed to ensure long-term spinal stability and maintenance of sagittal alignment. For details regarding these procedures, please refer to Chapter 7.

## Bony Anterior Column Injuries

*Injury Description*  Bony injuries of the subaxial anterior spinal column include all vertebral body fractures from C3 to C7. Chip fractures, longitudinal fractures, wedge compression fractures, and burst fractures are included in this group. Isolated injuries of this type are rare within the pediatric population. Fractures isolated to the anterior column are the most common fractures of the pediatric

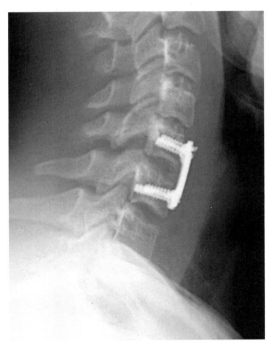

**Figure 4–8**    Postoperative lateral cervical spine film showing C5–C6 anterior cervical diskectomy and fusion with plating. Normal alignment is restored. This immediate postoperative film does not show solid arthrodesis between C5 and C6, but the patient ultimately went on to successful fusion.

subaxial spine.[68] These injuries are thought to be due to the higher concentration of collagen in younger intervertebral disks, making the disks less likely to rupture when subjected to traumatic stress. Axial loading and compressive forces are transmitted to the anulus fibrosus and on to the neighboring vertebral body, resulting in burst fractures or collapse. Denis outlined five subtypes of burst fractures: A, both end plates involved; B, superior end plate only; C, inferior end plate only; D, burst rotation; and E, burst lateral flexion.[69]

***Clinical Presentation***    Most patients present with neck pain related to their injury, although some patients may be asymptomatic on presentation. Most patients' injuries are discovered on the lateral cervical spine x-ray during a trauma evaluation at the hospital. In the event of an anterior column injury resulting in retropulsion of bony elements into the spinal canal or foramina, patients may present with myelopathy or radiculopathy. Higher cervical injuries are more likely to place patients at risk for spinal cord injury and are more frequent in younger children.

***Radiographic Diagnosis***    Almost all subaxial anterior spinal column fractures can be diagnosed by plain x-ray. Follow-up studies to evaluate the fracture further may include thin-cut CT scanning or MRI. For a comprehensive discussion of the radiology of these injuries, please refer to the classic text *The Radiology of Acute Cervical Spine Trauma*, by Harris and Edeiken-Monroe.[70] Once the anterior column has been compromised, one may see a decrease in vertebral body height and an increase in the interpedicular distance as well as splaying of the posterior joint surfaces. If these findings are absent on plain films and the index of suspicion is high enough for anterior column injury, CT should be performed. Anterior column fractures are often clearly delineated by reformatted CT imaging. If the mechanism of injury is severe enough or the patient's clinical exam is worrisome for spinal cord compression, MRI should be pursued. A retrospective analysis of 52 pediatric patients with a history of cervical trauma demonstrated the utility of MRI in identifying soft tissue injury, acute disk bulges, and longitudinal ligament disruption, all of which can influence the planning of surgical stabilization.[71] Furthermore, MRI can detect spinal cord contusions or infarctions after injuries characterized by minor, remote, or no fractures.[72]

In a study of cervical spine injuries in high-risk patients with multiple injuries, CT findings were compared with plain radiographs in detecting fracture and dislocations.[73] Plain radiography missed eight injuries (including three unstable injuries), and helical CT missed two. The respective sensitivity/specificity for plain radiographs and CT were 60%/100% and 90%/100%. Thus, in the setting of high-risk patients where cervical spine injury is suspected, CT scans are invaluable and should not be deferred.

***Treatment*** Anterior column injuries are often stable fractures and usually heal within 3 to 6 weeks. The most frequent form of treatment is conservative. Cervical collars are recommended for 2 to 4 weeks with follow-up flexion–extension films to confirm stability and absence of deformity.[68] The decision to treat anterior column injuries surgically in children is often motivated by kyphotic deformities generated by the fractures. Stable subaxial anterior spinal column fractures can be treated with a hard collar for a period of 1 to 2 months. Unstable injuries, including burst fractures with spinal cord compromise and fractures associated with significant ligamentous disruption, need to be managed surgically. Anterior cervical corpectomy and fusion with plating is the procedure of choice in those circumstances.

## Bony Posterior Column Injuries

***Injury Description*** Bony posterior column injuries include facet fractures, jumped or perched facets, lamina fractures, pedicle fractures, and spinous process fractures. Isolated bony posterior column injuries are rare in children and typically occur in combination with a posterior ligamentous injury. Unilateral and bilateral facet dislocations are likely the second most common injury to the pediatric cervical spine.[68] For example, it is assumed that in the cases of jumped facets, the capsular facet ligaments are torn and incompetent.

***Clinical Presentation*** Posterior column injuries often arise from hyperextension injuries, distraction injuries, or rotation shear injuries.[69] Almost all patients present with neck pain after trauma. Jumped or perched facets occur from a flexion–distraction mechanism, whereas facet complex impaction fractures are usually due to a rotation–compression mechanism. Lamina and spinous process fractures are often from hyperextension mechanisms. Isolated nerve root findings with neck pain are suspicious for a unilateral facet injury. Radicular and myelopathic neurological findings are not uncommon in this scenario.

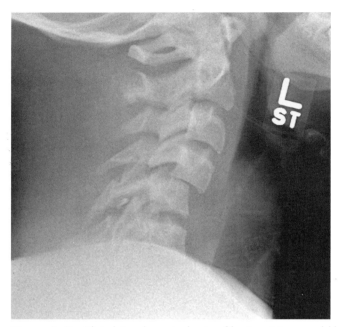

**Figure 4–9**   Plain lateral cervical spine film in a 14-year-old boy involved in a wrestling accident. The film shows 50% subluxation of C4 on C5, indicative of bilateral jumped facets.

***Radiographic Diagnosis***   Plain x-rays typically reveal jumped or perched facets and spinous process fractures, but other fractures of the posterior column are difficult to see without CT imaging. On plain film, subluxation greater than 50% of the vertebral body width is pathognomonic for bilateral jumped facets (**Fig. 4–9**). MRI will help determine if there is spinal cord injury or compression.

***Treatment***   Stable posterior column bony injuries can be treated with a cervical collar for comfort. Obviously unstable injuries, such as bilateral jumped facets, will need to be reduced and fused (**Fig. 4–10**). Closed reduction can be attempted manually or with tong traction, but it is prudent to obtain an MRI prior to reduction to rule out other pathology, such as a herniated disk, that might put the spinal cord at risk. If closed reduction fails, then open reduction as part of the fusion procedure is performed. Most of these injuries are handled from the posterior direction, the details of which are discussed in Chapter 7.

For other injuries, such as a unilateral perched or jumped facet, the decision as to whether the injury is stable or not is less clear. If the facet malposition can be corrected with closed reduction, the injury might heal itself over time. The amount of associated ligamentous injury and the involvement of the anterior column must be taken into account in making this decision. If conservative treatment is chosen, then it would be prudent to obtain a follow-up flexion–extension cervical spine film 2 to 3 months after the injury to determine if late stability is present. Of course, the presence of unremitting neck pain would more likely influence the decision toward surgical stabilization.

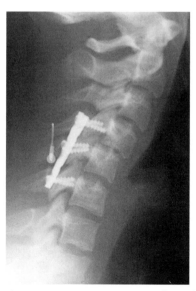

**Figure 4–10**   Postoperative lateral cervical spine film showing posterior plate and screw construct from C4 to C6, spanning the area of the bilateral jumped facets.

## Combined Anterior and Posterior Column Injuries

***Injury Description***   Combined anterior and posterior column injuries describe injury or disruption to all supporting structures of the cervical spine at one or more levels. They include, but are not limited to, injuries of the bones, ligaments, and soft tissue. Fracture dislocations, although rare in the pediatric age group, can occur, and are the focal point of this discussion. These injuries are discussed separately because of their severe nature and difficulty in management.

***Clinical Presentation***   Most patients present after severe trauma and have some element of neurological deficit from spinal cord injury; however, intact patients can be seen as well.

***Radiographic Diagnosis***   Plain films will show misalignment of the cervical spine, with perhaps distraction of the affected interspace (**Fig. 4–11**). CT will indicate if a fracture is part of the injury complex. MRI is particularly helpful, in that it clearly delineates the extent of the anterior and posterior column

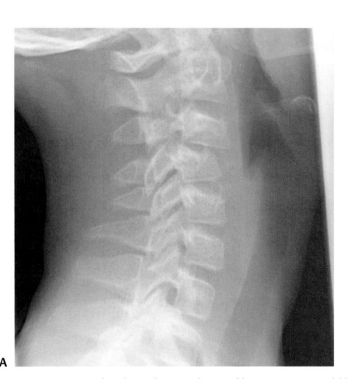
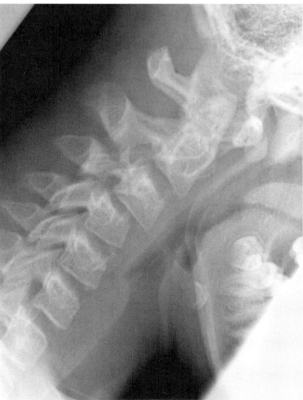

A

B

**Figure 4–11**   Plain lateral cervical spine film in a 12-year-old boy after trauma. Plain lateral cervical spine films in **(A)** extension and **(B)** flexion demonstrate subluxation of C3 on C4, with a maximal excursion of ~4 mm. Note a straightening of the normal cervical lordosis.

injuries (**Fig. 4–12**). Disk space rupture may result in a herniated disk fragment and must be noted prior to surgery.

***Treatment*** All injuries of this type must undergo surgical stabilization, by either an anterior or a posterior direction, or both. The goal of surgery is to both decompress the spinal canal of any bony elements in the spinal canal if necessary and provide columnar stability in a critically unstable region. Ideally, this should be performed within the first 12 to 48 hours. From the anterior direction, typically an anterior cervical diskectomy and fusion with plating is performed (**Fig. 4–13**). From the posterior direction, a rib-and-cable fusion, with or without instrumentation, is performed. It is recommended that in cases of gross cervical spine instability, a combined anterior and posterior fusion is performed to prevent hardware failure and avoid placement of halo orthosis.

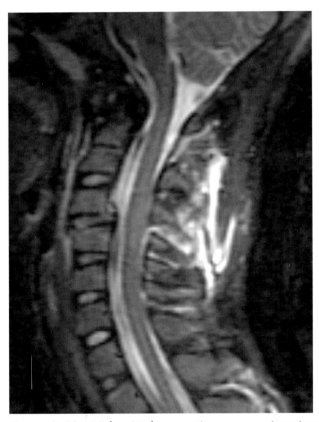

**Figure 4–12**    Midsagittal magnetic resonance imaging with short T1 inversion recovery sequence showing severe posterior ligamentous injury at C3–C4, with disk disruption at C3–C4 anteriorly and retropulsion of a disk fragment behind the body of C3.

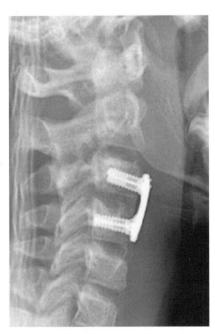

**Figure 4–13**    Postoperative plain lateral cervical spine film showing anterior cervical diskectomy at C3–C4 with realignment of the normal cervical lordosis. This patient was treated with an anterior construct alone. The patient ultimately achieved a solid bony arthrodesis between C3 and C4.

# ◆ Conclusion

The pediatric spine is not a scaled-down version of the adult spine. Injury patterns seen at the craniocervical junction in children are different from those seen in adults. Knowledge of developmental anatomy and a high index of suspicion are essential in the diagnosis and subsequent treatment of injuries in this area. Continued studies of injuries in this area are required to broaden our knowledge of the injury types seen, the consequences of those injuries, and the most appropriate treatments.

## References

1. Shulman ST, Madden JD, Esterly JR, Shanklin DR. Transection of spinal cord: a rare obstetrical complication of cephalic delivery. Arch Dis Child 1971;46: 291–294
2. Giguere JF, St-Vil D, Turmel A, et al. Airbags and children: a spectrum of C-spine injuries. J Pediatr Surg 1998;33:811–816
3. Adams VI. Neck injuries, II: Atlantoaxial dislocation: a pathologic study of 14 traffic fatalities. J Forensic Sci 1992;37:565–573
4. Bucholz RW, Burkhead WZ. The pathological anatomy of fatal atlanto-occipital dislocations. J Bone Joint Surg Am 1979;61:248–250
5. Dublin AB, Marks WM, Weinstock D, Newton TH. Traumatic dislocation of the atlanto-occipital articulation (AOA) with short-term survival: with a radiographic method of measuring the AOA. J Neurosurg 1980;52:541–546
6. Eismont FJ, Bohlman HH. Posterior atlanto-occipital dislocation with fractures of the atlas and odontoid process. J Bone Joint Surg Am 1978;60:397–399
7. Britt RH, Herrick MK, Mason RT, Dorfman LJ. Traumatic lesions of pontomedullary junction. Neurosurgery 1980;6:623–631
8. Lindenberg R, Freytag E. Brainstem lesions characteristic of traumatic hyperextension of the head. Arch Pathol 1970;90:509–515
9. Leestma JE, Kalelkar MB, Teas S. Ponto-medullary avulsion associated with cervical hyperextension. Acta Neurochir Suppl (Wien) 1983;32:69–73
10. Traynelis VC, Marano GD, Dunker RO, Kaufman HH. Traumatic atlanto-occipital dislocation: case report. J Neurosurg 1986;65:863–870
11. Grobovschek M, Scheibelbrandner W. Atlanto-occipital dislocation. Neuroradiology 1983;25:173–174
12. Gabrielsen TO, Maxwell JA. Traumatic atlanto-occipital dislocation: with case report of a patient who survived. Am J Roentgenol Radium Ther Nucl Med 1966;97:624–629
13. Pang D, Wilberger JE Jr. Traumatic atlanto-occipital dislocation with survival: case report and review. Neurosurgery 1980;7:503–508
14. Woodring JH, Selke AC Jr, Duff DE. Traumatic atlanto-occipital dislocation with survival. AJR Am J Roentgenol 1981;137:21–24
15. Montane I, Eismont FJ, Green BA. Traumatic occipitoatlantal dislocation. Spine 1991;16:112–116
16. Farley FA, Graziano GP, Hensinger RN. Traumatic atlanto-occipital dislocation in a child. Spine 1992;17:1539–1541

17. Matava MJ, Whitesides TE Jr, Davis PC. Traumatic atlanto-occipital dislocation with survival. Serial computerized tomography as an aid to diagnosis and reduction: a report of three cases. Spine 1993;18:1897–1903

18. Papadopoulos SM, Dickman CA, Sonntag VK, Rekate HL, Spetzler RF. Traumatic atlanto-occipital dislocation with survival. Neurosurgery 1991;28:574–579

19. Rockswold GL, Seljeskog EL. Traumatic atlantocranial dislocation with survival. Minn Med 1979;62:151–152, 154

20. Bools JC, Rose BS. Traumatic atlanto-occipital dislocation: two cases with survival. AJNR Am J Neuroradiol 1986;7:901–904

21. Collalto PM, DeMuth WW, Schwentker EP, Boal DK. Traumatic atlanto-occipital dislocation: case report. J Bone Joint Surg Am 1986;68:1106–1109

22. DiBenedetto T, Lee CK. Traumatic atlanto-occipital instability: a case report with follow-up and a new diagnostic technique. Spine 1990;15:595–597

23. Kaufman RA, Dunbar JS, Botsford JA, McLaurin RL. Traumatic longitudinal atlanto-occipital distraction injuries in children. AJNR Am J Neuroradiol 1982;3:415–419

24. Putnam WE, Stratton FT, Rohr RJ, Stitzell W, Roat G. Traumatic atlanto-occipital dislocations: value of the Powers ratio in diagnosis. J Am Osteopath Assoc 1986;86:798–804

25. Fruin AH, Pirotte TP. Traumatic atlanto-occipital dislocation: case report. J Neurosurg 1977;46:663–666

26. Georgopoulos G, Pizzutillo PD, Lee MS. Occipito-atlantal instability in children: a report of five cases and review of the literature. J Bone Joint Surg Am 1987;69:429–436

27. Powers B, Miller MD, Kramer RS, Martinez S, Gehweiler JA Jr. Traumatic anterior atlanto-occipital dislocation. Neurosurgery 1979;4:12–17

28. Altongy JF, Fielding JW. Combined atlanto-axial and occipito-atlantal rotatory subluxation: a case report. J Bone Joint Surg Am 1990;72:923–926

29. Clark CR, Kathol MH, Walsh T, el-Khoury GY. Atlantoaxial rotatory fixation with compensatory counter occipitoatlantal subluxation: a case report. Spine 1986;11:1048–1050

30. Watridge CB, Orrison WW, Arnold H, Woods GA. Lateral atlanto-occipital dislocation: case report. Neurosurgery 1985;17:345–347

31. Farthing J. Atlantocranial dislocation with survival: a case report. N C Med J 1948;9:34–36

32. Silbergeld DL, Laohaprasit V, Grady MS, Anderson PA, Winn HR. Two cases of fatal atlantoaxial distraction injury without fracture or rotation. Surg Neurol 1991;35:54–56

33. Anderson P, Montesano PX. Morphology and treatment of occipital condyle fractures. Spine 1988;13:731–736

34. Page CP, Story JL, Wissinger JP, Branch CL. Traumatic atlanto-occipital dislocation: case report. J Neurosurg 1973;39:394–397

35. Powers B, Miller MD, Kramer RS, et al. Traumatic anterior atlanto-occipital dislocation. Neurosurgery 1979;4:12–17

36. Pang D, Sahrakar K, Sun PP. Pediatric spinal cord and vertebral column injuries. In: Youmans JR, ed. Neurological Surgery: A Comprehensive Reference Guide to the Diagnosis and Management of Neurosurgical Problems. Vol 3. Philadelphia: WB Saunders; 1996:1991–2036

37. Birney TJ, Hanley EN Jr. Traumatic cervical spine injuries in childhood and adolescence. Spine 1989;14:1277–1282

38.  Fielding JW, Hawkins RJ, Hensinger RN, Francis WR. Atlantoaxial rotary deformities. Orthop Clin North Am 1978;9:955–967

39.  Phillips WA, Hensinger RN. The management of rotatory atlanto-axial subluxation in children. J Bone Joint Surg Am 1989;71:664–668

40.  Dyck P. Os odontoideum in children: neurological manifestations and surgical management. Neurosurgery 1978;2:93–99

41.  Fielding JW, Hawkins RJ. Atlanto-axial rotatory fixation. (Fixed rotatory subluxation of the atlanto-axial joint). J Bone Joint Surg Am 1977;59:37–44

42.  Bell C. The Nervous System of the Human Body. London: Longman, Rees, Orme, Brown and Green; 1830

43.  McGuire KJ, Silber J, Flynn JM, Levine M, Dormans JP. Torticollis in children: can dynamic computed tomography help determine severity and treatment? J Pediatr Orthop 2002;22:766–770

44.  Lee V, Pang D. Atlanto-axial rotatory fixation. In: Pang D, ed. Disorders of the Pediatric Spine. New York: Raven; 1995

45.  Hicazi A, Acaroglu E, Alanay A, Yazici M, Surat A. Atlantoaxial rotatory fixation-subluxation revisited: a computed tomographic analysis of acute torticollis in pediatric patients. Spine 2002;27:2771–2775

46.  Bohn D, Armstrong D, Becker L, Humphreys R. Cervical spine injuries in children. J Trauma 1990;30:463–469

47.  McGrory BJ, Klassen RA, Chao EY, Staeheli JW, Weaver AL. Acute fractures and dislocations of the cervical spine in children and adolescents. J Bone Joint Surg Am 1993;75:988–995

48.  Maiman DJ, Cusick JF. Traumatic atlantoaxial dislocation. Surg Neurol 1982;18:388–392

49.  Hamilton MG, Myles ST. Pediatric spinal injury: review of 61 deaths. J Neurosurg 1992;77:705–708

50.  Hadley MN, Zabramski JM, Browner CM, Rekate H, Sonntag VK. Pediatric spinal trauma: review of 122 cases of spinal cord and vertebral column injuries. J Neurosurg 1988;68:18–24

51.  Hill SA, Miller CA, Kosnik EJ, Hunt WE. Pediatric neck injuries: a clinical study. J Neurosurg 1984;60:700–706

52.  Fielding JW, Cochran GB, Lawsing JF III, Hohl M. Tears of the transverse ligament of the atlas: a clinical and biomechanical study. J Bone Joint Surg Am 1974;56:1683–1691

53.  Floman Y, Kaplan L, Elidan J, Umansky F. Transverse ligament rupture and atlanto-axial subluxation in children. J Bone Joint Surg Br 1991;73:640–643

54.  Locke GR, Gardner JI, Van Epps EF. Atlas-dens interval (ADI) in children: a survey based on 200 normal cervical spines. Am J Roentgenol Radium Ther Nucl Med 1966;97:135–140

55.  White AA, Panjabi MM. Clinical Biomechanics of the Spine. Philadelphia: JB Lippincott; 1990

56.  Dai L. Imaging diagnosis of cervical spine and spinal cord injuries in children. Chin J Traumatol 2001;4:222–225

57.  Dickman CA, Crawford NR, Paramore CG. Biomechanical characteristics of C1–2 cable fixations. J Neurosurg 1996;85:316–322

58.  Brockmeyer DL, York JE, Apfelbaum RI. Anatomical suitability of C1–2 transarticular screw placement in pediatric patients. J Neurosurg 2000;92(Suppl 1):7–11

59.  Lyon R. Pediatric spine injuries. In: Frymoyer JS, Wiesel SW, eds. The Adult and Pediatric Spine. Vol 1. Philadelphia: Lippincott Williams & Wilkins; 2004: 425–444

60. Eleraky MA, Theodore N, Adams M, Rekate HL, Sonntag VK. Pediatric cervical spine injuries: report of 102 cases and review of the literature. J Neurosurg 2000;92(Suppl 1):12–17

61. Mandabach M, Ruge JR, Hahn YS, McLone DG. Pediatric axis fractures: early halo immobilization, management and outcome. Pediatr Neurosurg 1993;19: 225–232

62. Sherk HH. Fractures of the atlas and odontoid process. Orthop Clin North Am 1978;9:973–984

63. Brockmeyer D, Apfelbaum R, Tippets R, Walker M, Carey L. Pediatric cervical spine instrumentation using screw fixation. Pediatr Neurosurg 1995;22: 147–157

64. Pizzutillo PD, Rocha EF, D'Astous J, Kling TF Jr, McCarthy RE. Bilateral fracture of the pedicle of the second cervical vertebra in the young child. J Bone Joint Surg Am 1986;68:892–896

65. Weiss MH, Kaufman B. Hangman's fracture in an infant. Am J Dis Child 1973;126:268–269

66. Finch GD, Barnes MJ. Major cervical spine injuries in children and adolescents. J Pediatr Orthop 1998;18:811–814

67. Pennecot GF, Leonard P, Peyrot Des Gachons S, Hardy JR, Pouliquen JC. Traumatic ligamentous instability of the cervical spine in children. J Pediatr Orthop 1984;4:339–345

68. Jones ET, Haid R. Injuries to the pediatric subaxial cervical spine. Semin Spine Surg 1991;3:61–70

69. Denis F. The three-column spine and its significance in the classification of acute thoracolumbar spinal injuries. Spine 1983;8:817–831

70. Harris JH Jr, Edeiken-Monroe B. The Radiology of Acute Cervical Spine Trauma. Philadelphia: Williams & Wilkins; 1986

71. Keiper MD, Zimmerman RA, Bilaniuk LT. MRI in the assessment of the supportive soft tissues of the cervical spine in acute trauma in children. Neuroradiology 1998;40:359–363

72. Davis PC, Reisner A, Hudgins PA, Davis WE, O'Brien MS. Spinal injuries in children: role of MR. AJNR Am J Neuroradiol 1993;14:607–617

73. Berne JD, Velmahos GC, El-Tawil Q, et al. Value of complete cervical helical computed tomographic scanning in identifying cervical spine injury in the unevaluable blunt trauma patient with multiple injuries: a prospective study. J Trauma 1999;47:896–903

# 5

# Advanced Atlantoaxial Surgery in Children

**Douglas L. Brockmeyer**

Atlantoaxial instability in any patient presents special challenges for the spinal surgeon, but these concerns are magnified in children. Small patient size, abnormal anatomy caused by craniovertebral anomalies, and a patient's growth potential are just some of the unique issues facing pediatric spine surgeons. Nevertheless, children demonstrate a very high capability for successful atlantoaxial arthrodesis.[1–8] This chapter outlines some of the key issues concerning atlantoaxial arthrodesis in children, including pertinent clinical findings, management strategies, and technical details concerning operative technique. One area of controversy in managing pediatric atlantoaxial instability concerns whether the risks of transarticular screw placement in the pediatric patient supersede the benefits of very high success rates when compared with previous methods of achieving fusion. This chapter does not seek to resolve that controversy but instead focuses on the technical aspects of safely performing successful atlantoaxial arthrodeses in children.

## ◆ Clinical Findings

Children with atlantoaxial instability present with several different types of symptoms. The most common presenting symptom is pain, which is present after almost every type of acute cervical traumatic accident severe enough to cause atlantoaxial instability. The pain is caused by stretching or disruption of the ligaments and muscles surrounding the atlantoaxial joint or by tearing of the bony periosteum following a fracture. Either way, persistent upper cervical spine pain following trauma is a very serious symptom that should be investigated thoroughly in children. Chronic cervical spine pain is more difficult to evaluate, and a complete medical history, including questions regarding remote trauma, must be obtained. Again, most children with chronic atlantoaxial instability will complain of some degree of cervical discomfort.

Torticollis is another common finding in children with atlantoaxial instability, especially when there is rotatory subluxation in the joint. The patient's torticollis may be painful or painless, depending on the etiology of the instability. Torticollis caused by acute trauma or an active, ongoing inflammatory process will cause a significant amount of discomfort. Children with painful torticollis may be very difficult to keep comfortable, even with significant amounts of analgesics. Painless torticollis is usually due to chronic atlantoaxial rotatory subluxation, os odontoideum, or a congenital vertebral anomaly. A complete radiographic evaluation, including plain cervical spine films and a thin-cut computed tomographic (CT) scan, should be undertaken in each child with painless torticollis to determine its exact etiology.[9]

Patients rarely present with neurological complaints such as weakness, numbness, or bladder incontinence. These findings are usually present only if there has been a significant trauma or long-standing, severe atlantoaxial instability causing spinal cord injury. The presence of a neurological deficit with atlantoaxial instability is an absolute indication for operative intervention.

General physical examination of the patient is often normal but may reflect findings associated with a congenital abnormality, such as Klippel-Feil syndrome (web neck, low-lying hairline, and limitation of neck motion), Down syndrome, or a systemic disorder such as cancer. Torticollis, scoliosis, and facial asymmetry are common findings associated with congenital anomalies. A small, dysmorphic stature may be found in a patient with skeletal dysplasia, including achondroplasia, spondyloepiphyseal dysplasia, and other metabolic forms of dwarfism.

Neurological signs, if present, mainly consist of myelopathy. Myelopathy presents as varying degrees of weakness or sensory disturbance in the upper or lower extremities. The myelopathy may mimic a "central cord syndrome" because of the preferential distribution of fibers subserving fine upper-extremity motor movement within the corticospinal tract.[10] Motor myelopathy is attributed to repetitive trauma of the pyramidal tracts and chronic compression of the spinal cord at the cervicomedullary junction.[11] Bladder disturbance tends to parallel the motor myelopathy. Sensory myelopathy is most often manifested by symptoms associated with posterior column dysfunction.

Vascular insufficiency may produce symptoms or signs associated with basilar migraines, syncope, vertigo, intermittent hemiparesis, altered consciousness, or transient visual field loss. These findings are rare but may be associated with compression or occlusion of the vertebral artery, anterior spinal artery, or perforating arteries of the spinal cord. The vascular-related symptoms or signs may be provoked by craniocervical rotation or angulation, often as a result of occult atlantoaxial instability.

# ◆ Management of Atlantoaxial Lesions

## Patient Evaluation

Not all patients with atlantoaxial abnormalities require surgery. Careful patient selection and application of conservative measures may save a patient from inappropriate surgery and its attendant risks.[12] Algorithms that deal with atlantoaxial problems may assist in the patient selection process (**Fig. 5–1**). The issues to be considered are the stability of the atlantoaxial joint, the reducibility of the lesion, the presence or absence of neurovascular compression, the natural history of the disease, and the growth potential of the patient. The stability of the atlantoaxial joint is the first concern in determining whether a patient will require operative stabilization. The atlantoaxial joint relies on the integrity of both the odontoid and the C2 transverse ligament for its stability.[13] If either of these structures is compromised, the joint is at risk for abnormal movement. Obviously, varying degrees of abnormal atlantoaxial movement can be tolerated. For example, it may be appropriate for a Down syndrome patient to demonstrate greater than normal atlantoaxial motion because of ligamentous

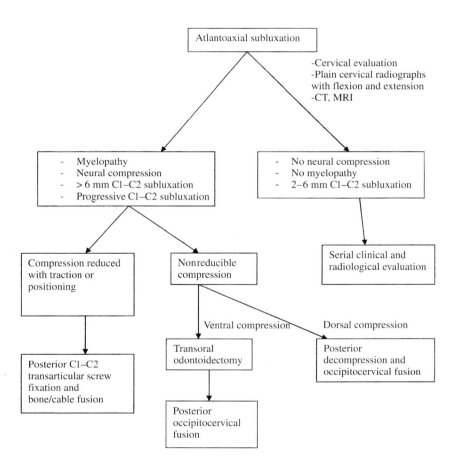

**Figure 5–1**   Algorithm for treatment of atlantoaxial instability.

laxity. There is a point, however, beyond which even seemingly benign atlantoaxial movement becomes dangerous. That point varies from patient to patient, and there are no fixed guidelines governing its existence. A general, well-accepted definition of abnormal atlantoaxial motion is an atlantodental interval (ADI) that measures greater than 4 mm. In 1984 the American Academy of Pediatrics arbitrarily chose an ADI greater than 4.5 mm as its cutoff for participation in the Special Olympics.[14] That decision has come under scrutiny from various authors, including the American Academy of Pediatrics,[15,16] and perhaps a less restrictive participation guideline is more appropriate.

An atlantoaxial abnormality may result in translation or rotatory subluxation of the joint. These abnormalities must be recognized and reduced as part of the treatment. Attempts at reduction can be performed with closed traction or, if that fails, open reduction. Neurovascular compression is also a very serious matter that must be managed with both joint stability and vascular integrity in mind. Occasionally, the timing of surgery is influenced by ongoing stroke therapy with either antiplatelet or anticoagulant agents.

The natural history of a given abnormality goes hand in hand with the patient's age and growth potential. For example, if a Down syndrome patient has a "stable" atlantoaxial joint documented by cervical spine flexion and extension films, it is known that this condition has a benign natural history.[16] That statement is true for patients approximately 10 years of age and older. There is little or no information concerning the natural history of atlantoaxial motion in patients younger than that age. Therefore, as a school-aged Down syndrome patient gets older, reexamination is only necessary if symptoms occur.[16] The algorithm shown in **Fig. 5–1** can be used to address issues with atlantoaxial instability in Down syndrome. Obviously, clinical judgment must be exercised in each case, but, generally, atlantoaxial laxity in Down syndrome does not deteriorate over time.

## Conservative Management

Various conditions of the atlantoaxial joint may be managed successfully in a conservative fashion. One of these conditions is atlantoaxial rotatory subluxation (AARS). AARS may be posttraumatic, postinfectious, or idiopathic in nature. AARS is typically managed in a stepwise fashion, with a cervical collar and oral antispasmodics as first-tier options, traction under sedation a second-tier option, and halo application under general anesthesia a third-tier option. Only severe, painful, refractory torticollis caused by AARS is managed with operative fusion.[17]

Another condition that may be managed successfully in a conservative fashion is os odontoideum. Currently, the appropriate management of asymptomatic patients with os odontoideum and no neurological signs is controversial, although it is generally agreed that patients with symptoms or signs should undergo operative intervention. The Guidelines for the Management of Acute Cervical Spine and Spinal Cord Injuries[18] found that there was insufficient evidence to support standards or guidelines in the diagnosis or management of os odontoideum. As an option, the authors suggested that asymptomatic patients with os odontoideum may be managed conservatively. We believe, however, that the lifelong risks associated with an untreated os odontoideum in an active pediatric patient, such as potential high cervical spinal cord injury or progressive instability, outweigh the risks associated with surgical stabilization. In our series of 24 patients with os odontoideum, all patients underwent C1–C2 transarticular screw fixation without any surgical morbidity, and all had successful fusion within 4 months without a halo orthosis.

Another group of patients with atlantoaxial instability who may not require surgery, at least initially, is the very young. Very young patients (2 years of age or less) are generally managed with a custom-fitted external orthosis to provide protection and support until the patient is old enough to undergo safe operative management. Even in very young patients, however, as instrumentation and surgical techniques improve, it may be possible to provide operative stability in selected cases that obviously require fusion (**Figs. 5–2** and **5–3**). As time goes

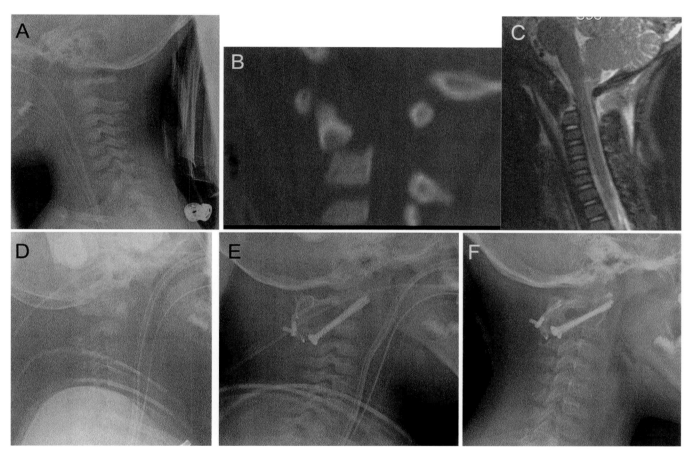

**Figure 5–2**    A 22-month-old girl with an odontoid synchondrosis fracture following a motor vehicle accident. **(A)** Preoperative lateral cervical spine film showing fracture through the C2 odontoid synchondrosis. **(B)** Midsagittal reconstruction showing the odontoid synchondrosis fracture, with angulation and anterior subluxation of the fracture fragment. **(C)** Midsagittal T2-weighted magnetic resonance imaging scan showing high signal intensity in the posterior ligamentous and muscular structure, indicative of C1–C2 instability. **(D)** Lateral cervical spine film of the patient in halo, demonstrating that angulation and anterior subluxation are still present. **(E)** Early postoperative lateral cervical spine film showing placement of C1–C2 transarticular screws and posterior bone-and-cable fusion in "girth-hitch" style. **(F)** Follow-up film of this patient obtained 4 years postsurgery showing solid bony arthrodesis between the posterior elements of C1 and C2. Note the absence of any spinal deformity or juxtafusion pathology.

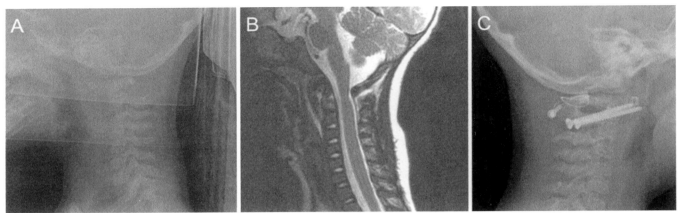

**Figure 5–3** An 18-month-old girl with Down syndrome and atlantoaxial instability. **(A)** Preoperative lateral cervical spine film showing atlantoaxial subluxation. **(B)** Preoperative T2-weighted sagittal magnetic resonance imaging showing craniocervical narrowing. **(C)** Postoperative lateral cervical spine film showing C1–C2 transarticular screws and solid arthrodesis between the posterior atlantoaxial area.

on, the strategies and techniques used to manage this extremely challenging patient population will improve.

## Surgical Management and Decision Making

The decision to proceed with surgery in a patient with atlantoaxial instability is based on several issues. The amount of atlantoaxial motion that is present is an obvious factor. Traditional teaching dictates that an ADI greater than 4.5 mm on a flexion x-ray indicates excess atlantoaxial motion. A more direct measurement relating to atlantoaxial instability is the neural canal width (NCW). An NCW less than 12 mm correlates with spinal cord compression and is further evidence of atlantoaxial instability.[19]

Patient age is also an important factor. Some authors have discounted the placement of transarticular screws in any pediatric patient, citing the high risk of potential complications in that population,[5] or have stated that the lowest appropriate age for C1–C2 transarticular screw fixation should be 4 or 5 years.[20] A recent publication by our group[21] has redefined previously held notions regarding the lowest age in which C1–C2 transarticular screws can be placed successfully. The youngest patient in our series was 18 months old. We have safely placed 24 C1–C2 transarticular screws in 13 patients 4 years of age or younger (19% of our overall series), providing evidence that transarticular screw fixation of the atlantoaxial joint is safe and effective in this very young age group. Further follow-up is necessary to determine the long-term effects of C1–C2 transarticular screw placement, but our initial experience is very encouraging. After following 10 of our young atlantoaxial fusion patients for at least 4 years, we have not seen any significant adverse effects.

Size-for-age constraints may also be encountered in patients with atlantoaxial pathology. For example, a 12-year-old patient with Morquio's syndrome may have a vertebral column the size of a normal 5-year-old child.

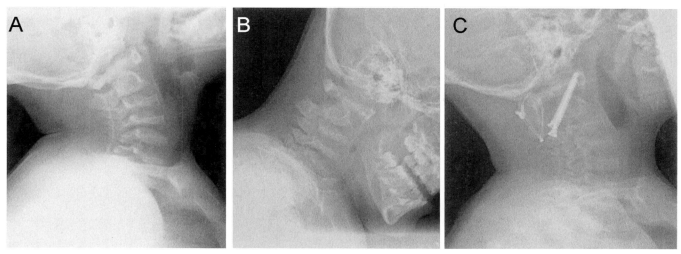

**Figure 5–4**   A 4-year-old boy with metatrophic dwarfism, hypoplastic dens, and atlantoaxial instability. **(A)** Preoperative lateral cervical spine film, with patient in extension. **(B)** Preoperative lateral cervical spine film, with patient in flexion. Note significant presence of atlantoaxial instability. **(C)** Postoperative lateral cervical spine film showing placement of C1–C2 transarticular screws and posterior bone-and-cable fusion with solid arthrodesis.

Therefore, the surgeon must be comfortable working with smaller patients and the distorted anatomy that may be encountered. These anatomical challenges may be extreme, as seen in **Fig. 5–4**.

## Surgical Approaches

The vast majority of atlantoaxial fusion procedures are performed through a midline posterior incision extending from the suboccipital area to the midcervical region. Anterior cervical approaches for odontoid screw fixation are used frequently and are well described in adults or adult-sized patients.[22] There are two reports of pediatric patients who have undergone odontoid screw fixation, but the procedure is not commonly performed in children.[8] It is not the aim of this chapter to review procedures that are uncommonly performed in children, including odontoid screw fixation and other more esoteric procedures such as direct anterior atlantoaxial screw fixation. For general purposes, posterior midline procedures and their variations are best when dealing with pediatric patients and immature spinal anatomy.

## Implants

Several different techniques for posterior atlantoaxial fusion have been described in the literature over the years. Among these, the Gallie– and Sonntag–style fusions have become the most popular.[23,24] These fusions are supplemented either by an external halo orthosis or by a hard cervical collar.

When performing an atlantoaxial fusion, the bone graft is most often harvested from the posterior iliac crest. Occasionally, in very young patients or in patients where the iliac crest is absent or unsuitable, rib graft is harvested. We have described a "girth-hitch" atlantoaxial fusion using rib grafts in patients 2 years of age or less.[25] In the Gallie, Sonntag, or girth-hitch constructs, the bone graft is held in place by a thin titanium multistranded cable (Songer cable, Medtronic Sofamor Danek, Memphis, TN).

C1–C2 transarticular screws, initially described by Grob and Magerl in 1987,[26] are now a well-accepted way of providing immediate stability to the atlantoaxial joint. Most experience with this technique has been described in adults;[27–31] however, there are several case series describing the use of this technique in children.[1,2,8] C1–C2 transarticular screws, if chosen, are typically fully threaded titanium implants in either a 3.5 or 4.0 mm outer diameter (OD). To place a 4.0 mm OD screw, a 3.0 mm drill followed by a 3.5 mm tap is used. To place a 3.5 mm OD screw, the 3.0 mm drill is used, and the screw is placed without tapping the hole to obtain sufficient purchase in the bone.

Biomechanical considerations for posterior atlantoaxial fusions are important. Adequate restriction of motion in the rotational, translational, and flexion–extension planes is critical to creating an optimal environment for bony fusion to occur. If C1–C2 transarticular screw fixation and posterior bone-and-cable fusion are chosen for the arthrodesis, all significant planes of motion are prevented. The transarticular screws prevent motion in the rotational and translational planes, whereas the posterior construct prevents motion in flexion and extension. If transarticular screws are not placed, and an external halo orthosis is used instead, it is not nearly as efficient in preventing rotation and translation at the atlantoaxial level. This may explain why fusion results with a bone-and-wire construct with halo arthrodesis were in the 90% range in a large adult series[24] and 84% in a pediatric series.[5] In contrast, fusion results with a Sonntag construct and C1–C2 transarticular screws were 100% in two pediatric series.[8,21]

## Bone Graft Materials

As already mentioned, posterior iliac crest is used as the grafting material in the majority of patients undergoing atlantoaxial fusion. Other options include allograft, rib graft, or either split-thickness or full-thickness suboccipital bone. Because a posterior atlantoaxial graft (such as a Sonntag-style fusion) is in place under tension in a semi-interbody position, allograft can be used successfully, although there is not much experience in using it in this way. Further work regarding the use of allograft bone in this surgical technique is necessary. For very young patients (< 3 years old), we place autologous rib graft fastened with a girth-hitch fusion technique.[25] With the girth-hitch fusion and C1–C2 transarticular screw fixation, two patients under 3 years of age had successful atlantoaxial fusion. The use of suboccipital bone for atlantoaxial fusion has been described and has been used with some success.[3]

## External Orthoses

External orthoses include soft and hard cervical collars, halo braces, sterno-occipital mandibular immobilization (SOMI) braces, and custom occipitothoracic devices. Each device has specific indications for use. Cervical collars are generally used for protection of spinal alignment following trauma, for pain relief, and to aid in the healing of stable cervical spine fractures. Halo and SOMI orthoses are generally used after spine fusion surgery to maintain spinal alignment and provide primary support of a bony fusion construct or secondary support to an internal fixation device. They might also be used as a primary way to heal unstable cervical spine fractures, such as an odontoid synchondrosis fracture in a young patient or a type II odontoid fracture in a teenager. Either way, external orthoses are imperfect systems that rely on semirigid materials and fixation points to provide spinal stability. Not surprisingly, multiple case series report lower fusion rates when using halo orthoses versus direct methods of screw fixation for an unstable joint.[5,32,33] We have currently limited our practice in placing halo devices to two circumstances: (1) management of C2 odontoid synchondrosis fractures and (2) supplementation of internal fixation postoperatively when spinal fixation is tenuous or the degree of preoperative instability is extreme.

## ◆ Postoperative Follow-up

### Radiographic Protocol

Once a posterior atlantoaxial fusion procedure has been performed, it is paramount that the surgeon follows the patient long enough to document whether a successful arthrodesis has been achieved. For children, this is usually 3 to 4 months. A plain lateral cervical spine film is sufficient to determine whether a successful fusion is present. Attention to the bone graft between the posterior arch of C1 and the posterior elements of C2 should reveal well-corticated bridging bone between those two structures. Our protocol at Primary Children's Medical Center calls for monthly plain lateral cervical spine films until the patient fuses. Occasionally, a thin-cut CT scan with two-dimensional reconstructions is necessary to evaluate the status of the fusion more closely.

### Failed Fusions

Ten patients have been referred to our institution following failed fusion attempts. Our experience has shown that most failed atlantoaxial fusions have resulted either from a failure to use a proper method of rigid internal fixation or from an improperly applied arthrodesis. If rigid internal fixation has not been used previously, we place direct screw fixation and instrumentation at the appropriate level. We then revise the fusion using autograft and remove the halo, if one has been placed.

### Postoperative Growth Potential

The patient's postoperative growth potential or potential for spinal deformity is a source of concern for many pediatric surgeons. It has been shown that pediatric cervical spine growth potential after ~10 years of age is very small.[34,35]

With younger patients, however, more careful analysis is required. In our 10-year experience with rigid screw fixation constructs in over 50 pediatric patients age 18 months to 16 years, "growth arrest" occurs once the patient achieves successful fusion at the atlantoaxial level. If the bone in the area of fusion subsequently grows a small amount, it remodels around the hardware, and no cranioverterbral deformity is seen. Therefore, we believe that posterior C1–C2 screw fixation and fusion may be routinely performed in children as young as ~2 to 3 years. The anatomical suitability of younger patients must be evaluated on a case by case basis.

Parisini et al[36] found no sagittal cervical deformity 12 months after C1–C2 fusion in a series of pediatric patients. Our experience has been similar. Even in our youngest patients, no growth deformity in either the sagittal or coronal plane has been noted on multiple postoperative imaging studies, some measuring out over 5 years. It is our opinion that future growth potential and risk of deformity are important, but they have not turned out to be significant concerns in this patient population when compared with the risk of untreated atlantoaxial or cranioverterbral instability.

## ◆ An Advanced Technique for Atlantoaxial Arthrodesis

We will now focus on the operative technique of performing C1–C2 transarticular screw fixation in children. This procedure is technically very demanding and requires an intimate knowledge of the atlantoaxial joint and its surroundings. In children, it has the additional demands of dealing with congenital vertebral anomalies and size-for-age constraints in patients with dwarfism or metabolic bone disorders. Our protocol for patients with atlantoaxial instability is to proceed with C1–C2 transarticular screw fixation and bone-and-cable fusion without a halo, except in very young patients with C2 synchondrosis fractures. For patients with C2 synchondrosis fractures, we initially manage them in a halo and proceed with surgery only if the halo fails to hold their reduction.

Once the decision to proceed with atlantoaxial stabilization with C1–C2 transarticular screws has been made, the preoperative planning phase begins. The planning phase consists of two phases: (1) imaging and image analysis, and (2) screw placement strategies.

### Imaging and Image Analysis

At a minimum, our preoperative imaging protocol consists of plain cervical spine films with flexion and extension, along with thin-cut (1 mm) axial CT scans from occiput to C3 with two-dimensional sagittal and coronal reconstructions. No presurgical flexion–extension films are obtained in trauma patients with obviously unstable fractures of the atlantoaxial segments. Magnetic resonance imaging (MRI) is helpful in some cases but not critical in the planning phase for placing C1–C2 transarticular screws. Image analysis of the thin-cut CT section is performed on a high-speed CT workstation. Multiplanar reconstructions in the screw trajectory pathway are generated to determine the best path for screw placement.[2]

At this stage, a decision is made regarding what size screw, if any, should be placed on each side of the patient in question. In general, we use 3.5 mm OD screws for patients 4 years of age and younger and 4.0 mm OD screws for patients older than 4 years. Each case is unique, however, and the screw diameter appropriate for each patient should be determined only after careful study of the reformatted images.

Before surgery, we also have a clear understanding of the anatomical landmarks essential in determining the starting point for screw trajectory. The screw starting point is measured in millimeters from the midportion of the C2–C3 facet joint. The screw trajectory is defined in number of degrees from both the parasagittal plane and the dorsal or ventral position of the screw relative to the vertebral artery foramen in C2.

## Screw Placement Strategies

If it is determined during the preoperative planning that one side is unsafe for transarticular screw placement, other strategies must be considered. For patients with atlantoaxial instability and only one safe transarticular screw pathway, a unilateral C1–C2 transarticular screw is placed, followed by an autograft bone-and-cable fusion. Four patients in our study[21] underwent unilateral C1–C2 transarticular screw fixation for atlantoaxial instability. They all went on to achieve successful fusion. We encountered no patients with atlantoaxial instability in whom at least one C1–C2 transarticular screw could not be placed safely. Another strategy in this situation would be to place a "Harms-style" construct on the side in question.[37] The Harms construct consists of a C1 lateral mass screw and C2 pars screw connected by a top-loading rod system. There is, however, very little experience with this technique in the pediatric population.

We believe the preoperative planning phase is critical to avoiding injury of the vertebral artery during C1–C2 transarticular screw placement.[2] If at any time the fluoroscopic data do not match the preoperative CT data and what is seen during surgery, we elect not to place the transarticular screw. Generally, we start on the "safest side" to place a screw so that at least one good screw is inserted as part of the construct. If the vertebral artery is injured during placement of the first screw, the screw is placed to tamponade bleeding, and placement of the second screw is abandoned. Postoperatively, the patient undergoes a vertebral angiogram to assess whether an arterial injury, such as a pseudoaneurysm, has been formed. On the angiogram, thrombosis of the entire vertebral artery on the affected side is usually seen, with the distal end of the thrombosis at the junction of the contralateral vertebral artery and the basilar artery. If the vertebral artery is injured during placement of the second screw (placed only if no injury is encountered with the first screw), the screw is placed as usual. The same postoperative imaging protocol is used as already described.

After the preoperative planning phase is over, the patient is taken to the operating room (**Fig. 5–5**). A few brief comments regarding the room setup and patient positioning are appropriate here. We do not routinely use spinal cord monitoring as part of this procedure. Once the patient is intubated (either with

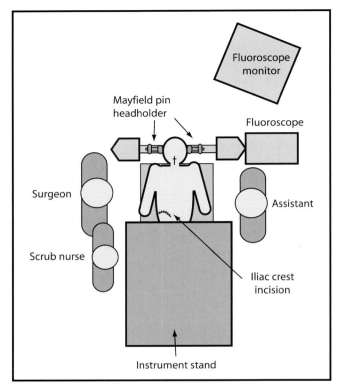

**Figure 5–5**    Operating room setup for C1–C2 transarticular screw fixation.

axial traction or with a hard collar in place), the patient is lifted and turned carefully in axial alignment into the prone position.

Mayfield three-point fixation is routinely used in all patients, even in patients as young as 2 years of age. Gentle axial traction is applied (except in cases of atlanto-occipital dislocation) under direct lateral fluoroscopic vision, and then the patient's neck is flexed and posteriorly translated into the "military tuck" position (**Fig. 5–6**). All manipulations of the cervical spine are done with direct fluoroscopic guidance. We do not use intraoperative stereotactic navigation. We believe the reference arc currently available for commercial use in stereotactic spine navigation is awkward, cumbersome, and prone to error when attached to the spinous process of a young child. Instead, we prefer to use the preoperative CT images correlated with the intraoperative fluoroscopic information to place the transarticular screws.

A midline upper cervical and lower suboccipital incision is marked out, along with two upper thoracic paramedian incisions (**Fig. 5–7**). The midline

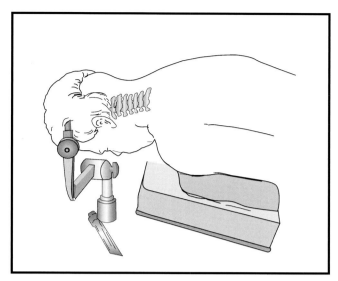

**Figure 5–6**   Patient position with head held by headholder. Neck is placed in military tuck position.

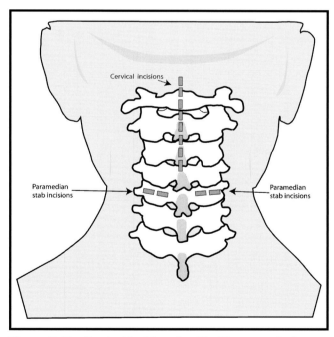

**Figure 5–7**   Cervical incisions for C1–C2 transarticular screw fixation.

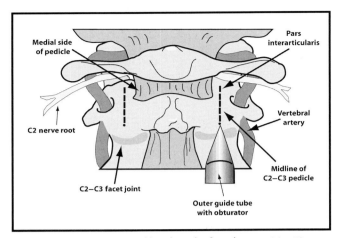

**Figure 5–8**   Anatomical landmarks for placing C1–C2 transarticular screws.

incision is opened, and the paraspinous musculature is dissected laterally. The posterior C1, C2, and upper C3 complex is exposed, and the C2 pedicle is skeletonized medially and laterally so that its borders are clearly identified (**Fig. 5–8**). One of the upper thoracic paramedian incisions is opened, and the outer guide tube with soft tissue obturator is passed through it into the cervical incision site (**Fig. 5–9A**). The obturator is removed, and an awl is passed through the outer guide tube. Using the awl, a starting hole corresponding to the entry point of the transarticular screw is placed near the midline of the C2-C3 facet joint. The awl is withdrawn and replaced with an inner guide tube (**Fig. 5–9B**). A 3.0 mm OD drill bit (with drill attached) is passed down the inner tube, and its tip is placed in the pilot hole. Using fluoroscopic guidance, a hole is drilled through the C2 lamina, C2 pedicle, C2 pars interarticularis, C1–C2 interspace, and C1 lateral mass sequentially (**Fig. 5–9C**). The target point for the drill is typically the midportion of the C1 anterior arch (**Fig. 5–9D**). The drill and inner guide tube are removed, and the hole is tapped with a 3.5 mm outer diameter tap (**Fig. 5–9E**). The tap is withdrawn, and a 4.0 mm outer diameter screw of proper length is then placed through the tapped hole (**Fig. 5–9F**). A C1–C2 interspinous bone-and-cable fusion is placed using a posterior iliac crest bone graft (**Fig. 5–10**).

For patients with a rotatory component to their C1–C2 instability, the C1–C2 rotation often cannot be reduced before surgery. If that is the case, the posterior C1–C2 interspace assumes a trapezoidal configuration at surgery (**Fig. 5–11A**). Placing a transarticular screw through the C1–C2 interspace is dangerous in that circumstance because the C1–C2 joint does not align properly. To remedy the situation, the C1–C2 joint can be reduced by applying gentle distraction and rotation to the head during surgery. This maneuver must be performed under direct fluoroscopic guidance. Once the C1–C2 joint is realigned, the C1–C2 interspace should assume a rectangular appearance (**Fig. 5–11B**). It is now safe to proceed with placing C1–C2 transarticular screws.

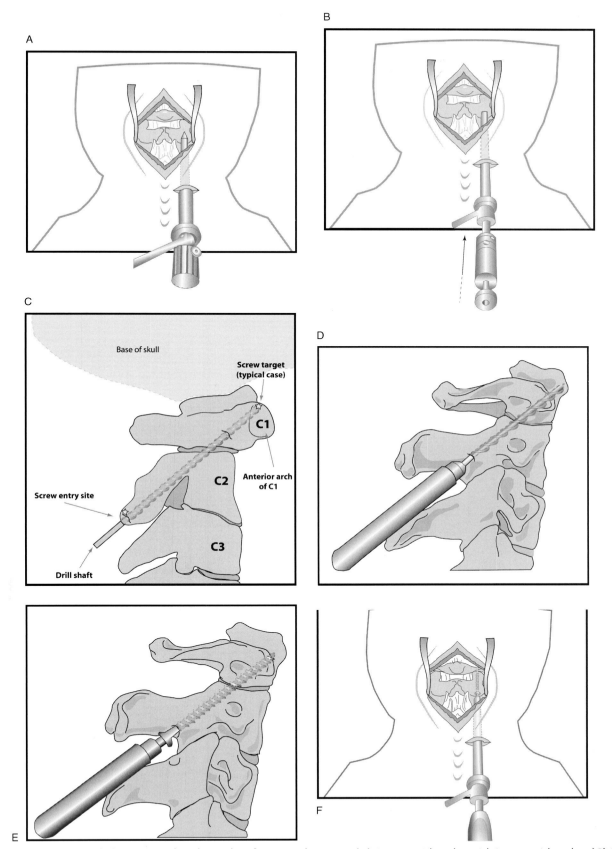

**Figure 5–9** **(A)** Outer guide tube with soft tissue obturator. **(B)** Outer guide tube with inner guide tube. **(C)** Screw trajectory seen in lateral fluoroscopic view. **(D)** Lateral view of drill. **(E)** Lateral view of tap. **(F)** Top view of screw placement.

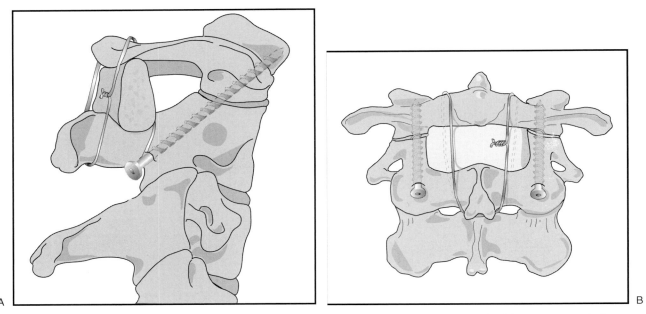

**Figure 5–10** **(A)** Lateral and **(B)** anteroposterior views of final construct with bone-and-cable Sonntag-style fusion.

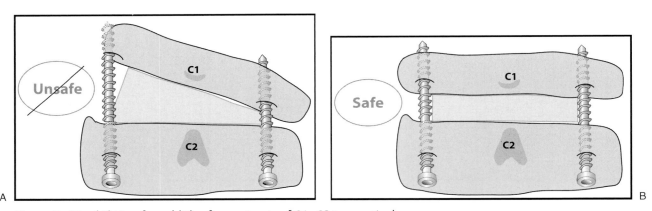

**Figure 5–11** **(A)** Unsafe and **(B)** safe constructs of C1–C2 transarticular screws.

### References

1. Brockmeyer D, Apfelbaum R, Tippets R, Walker M, Carey L. Pediatric cervical spine instrumentation using screw fixation. Pediatr Neurosurg 1995;22: 147–157

2. Brockmeyer DL, York JE, Apfelbaum RI. Anatomical suitability of C1–2 transarticular screw placement in pediatric patients. J Neurosurg 2000;92(Suppl 1):7–11

3. Casey AT, Hayward RD, Harkness WF, Crockard HA. The use of autologous skull bone grafts for posterior fusion of the upper cervical spine in children. Spine 1995;20:2217–2220

4. Kumar R, Nayak SR. Management of pediatric congenital atlantoaxial dislocation: a report of 23 cases from northern India. Pediatr Neurosurg 2002;36: 197–208

5. Lowry DW, Pollack IF, Clyde B, Albright AL, Adelson PD. Upper cervical spine fusion in the pediatric population. J Neurosurg 1997;87:671–676

6. Sawin PD, Traynelis VC, Menezes AH. A comparative analysis of fusion rates and donor-site morbidity for autogeneic rib and iliac crest bone grafts in posterior cervical fusions. J Neurosurg 1998;88:255–265

7. Schultz KD Jr, Petronio J, Haid RW, et al. Pediatric occipitocervical arthrodesis: a review of current options and early evaluation of rigid internal fixation techniques. Pediatr Neurosurg 2000;33:169–181

8. Wang J, Vokshoor A, Kim S, Elton S, Kosnik E, Bartkowski H. Pediatric atlantoaxial instability: management with screw fixation. Pediatr Neurosurg 1999;30: 70–78

9. Pang D, Li V. Atlantoaxial rotatory fixation, I: Biomechanics of normal rotation at the atlantoaxial joint in children. Neurosurgery 2004;55:614–626

10. Levi AD, Tator CH, Bunge RP. Clinical syndromes associated with disproportionate weakness of the upper versus the lower extremities after cervical spinal cord injury. Neurosurgery 1996;38:179–183

11. Dickman C, Hadley M, Pappas C. Cruciate paralysis: a clinical and radiographic analysis of injuries to the cervicomedullary junction. J Neurosurg 1990;73: 850–858

12. Rockswold GL, Bergman TA, Ford SE. Halo immobilization and surgical fusion: relative indications and effectiveness in the treatment of 140 cervical spine injuries. J Trauma 1990;30:893–898

13. White AA, Panjabi MM. The clinical biomechanics of the occipitoatlantoaxial complex. Orthop Clin North Am 1978;9:867–878

14. American Academy of Pediatrics. Committee on Sports Medicine: atlantoaxial instability in Down syndrome. Pediatrics 1984;74:152–154

15. American Academy of Pediatrics Committee on Sports Medicine and Fitness. Atlantoaxial instability in Down syndrome: subject review. Pediatrics 1995;96 (Pt 1):151–154

16. Brockmeyer D. Down syndrome and craniovertebral instability: topic review and treatment recommendations. Pediatr Neurosurg 1999;31:71–77

17. Crossman JE, David K, Hayward R, Crockard HA. Open reduction of pediatric atlantoaxial rotatory fixation: long-term outcome study with functional measurements. J Neurosurg 2004;100:235–240

18. Os odontoideum. Neurosurgery 2002;50(Suppl 3):S148–S155

19. White KS, Ball WS, Prenger EC, Patterson BJ, Kirks DR. Evaluation of the craniocervical junction in Down syndrome: correlation of measurements obtained with radiography and MR imaging. Radiology 1993;186:377–382

20. Rekate HL, Theodore N, Sonntag VK, Dickman CA. Pediatric spine and spinal cord trauma: state of the art for the third millennium. Childs Nerv Syst 1999;15:743–750

21. Gluf WM, Brockmeyer DL. Atlantoaxial transarticular screw fixation: a review of surgical indications, fusion rate, complications, and lessons learned in 67 pediatric patients. J Neurosurg Spine 2005;2:164–169

22. Apfelbaum RI, Lonser RR, Veres R, Casey A. Direct anterior screw fixation for recent and remote odontoid fractures. J Neurosurg 2000;93(Suppl 2):227–236

23. Gallie WE. Fracture and dislocations of the cervical spine. Am J Surg 1939;46: 495–499

24. Dickman CA, Sonntag VK, Papadopoulos SM, Hadley MN. The interspinous method of posterior atlantoaxial arthrodesis. J Neurosurg 1991;74:190–198

25. Brockmeyer DL. A bone and cable girth-hitch technique for atlantoaxial fusion in pediatric patients. J Neurosurg 2002;97:400–402

26. Grob D, Magerl F. Surgical stabilization of C1 and C2 fractures. Orthopade 1987;16:46–54

27. Grob D, Jeanneret B, Aebi M, Markwalder TM. Atlanto-axial fusion with transarticular screw fixation. J Bone Joint Surg Br 1991;73:972–976

28. Haid RW Jr, Subach BR, McLaughlin MR, Rodts GE Jr, Wahlig JB Jr. C1–C2 transarticular screw fixation for atlantoaxial instability: a 6-year experience. Neurosurgery 2001;49:65–68 discussion 69–70

29. Apfelbaum R. Posterior C1–2 screw fixation for atlantoaxial instability. In: Rengachary SS, Wilkins RH, eds. Neurosurgical Operative Atlas. Vol 4, no. 1. Baltimore: Williams & Wilkins; 1995:19–28

30. Apfelbaum RI. Posterior transarticular C1–2 screw fixation for atlantoaxial instability. Aesculap Scientific Information 1994;25:1–4

31. Dickman CA, Sonntag VK. Posterior C1–C2 transarticular screw fixation for atlantoaxial arthrodesis. Neurosurgery 1998;43:275–281

32. Moon MS, Choi WT, Moon YW, Moon JL, Kim SS. Brooks' posterior stabilisation surgery for atlantoaxial instability: review of 54 cases. J Orthop Surg (Hong Kong) 2002;10:160–164

33. Lennarson PJ, Mostafavi H, Traynelis VC, Walters BC. Management of type II dens fractures: a case-control study. Spine 2000;25:1234–1237

34. Sherk H, Nicholson J, Chung S. Fractures of the odontoid process in young children. J Bone Joint Surg Am 1978;60:921–924

35. Bailey D. The normal cervical spine in infants and children. Radiology 1952;69:712–719

36. Parisini P, Di Silvestre M, Greggi T, Bianchi G. C1–C2 posterior fusion in growing patients: long-term follow-up. Spine 2003;28:566–572 discussion 572

37. Harms J, Melcher RP. Posterior C1–C2 fusion with polyaxial screw and rod fixation. Spine 2001;26:2467–2471

# 6

# Advanced Occipitocervical Surgery in Children

**Douglas L. Brockmeyer**

In general, anomalies of the craniovertebral junction (CVJ) can be divided into three main categories: congenital, developmental, and acquired. For purposes of simplicity and clarity, developmental and acquired anomalies are often placed under the same heading.

Congenital CVJ anomalies are those that are present at birth and remain relatively static over time. Their presence ultimately may lead to clinical instability and require treatment. Common examples of such anomalies include occipitalization of the atlas, basilar invagination, and segmentation failure of C1–C2 or C2–C3. Developmental anomalies are those that arise out of an ongoing pathological process that directly affects the CVJ, such as Down syndrome, Klippel-Feil syndrome, and osteogenesis imperfecta. Acquired anomalies arise as part of a systemic disease, infection, inflammation, or trauma. Examples include traumatic atlanto-occipital dislocation, rheumatoid arthritis, and osteomyelitis.

A surgical physiological approach to CVJ problems has been proposed by Menezes.[1] He argues that several factors must be taken into account for a complete understanding of a given anomaly: (1) the reducibility of the lesion; (2) the direction and manner of the encroachment of the lesion, along with neurological deficits; (3) lesion etiology (e.g., bony versus soft tissue, intracranial versus extracranial, intramedullary versus extramedullary); and (4) the growth potential of the affected area. Stability of the CVJ is paramount. Reducible lesions require reduction prior to operative stabilization, whereas an irreducible lesion may be fused in situ. Postoperative stabilization may be necessary for mass lesions requiring enough bone or ligament removal to cause instability. This chapter reviews the clinical presentation of children with CVJ abnormalities, discusses the surgical and nonsurgical management of these disorders, and presents a detailed discussion of newer techniques of craniocervical instrumentation.

# ◆ Clinical Findings

The clinical findings that result from disorders of the CVJ are diverse and reflect the densely packed ascending and descending fiber tracts, brain stem nuclei, and cranial nerves that reside within this region. Each CVJ abnormality varies in its degree of bony or soft tissue deformity, its clinical effects on neurovascular structures, and its associated effects on adjacent skeletal anatomy. Therefore, individual patients present with their own constellation of clinical findings. These findings may result from compression or compromise of the lower brain stem, cervical spinal cord, cranial nerves, or vascular structures and may have secondary effects such as progressive herniation, syringohydromyelia formation, or hydrocephalus.

The most common presenting symptom is pain, which may be manifested by headache or neck discomfort. Suboccipital headache may be caused by irritation of the second cervical nerve as it passes through the atlantoaxial joint capsule. Localized neck pain is most commonly attributed to destruction or disruption of periosteal or soft tissue structures brought about by the disease process. Other symptoms are most often a part of specific neurological or vascular syndromes.

Symptoms may progress insidiously and may present with false localizing signs.[2] In some rare instances, the patient may present with catastrophic neurological deterioration or even sudden death. A history of a minor antecedent trauma resulting in rather rapid neurological decline is not uncommon.[2]

General physical examination of the patient is often normal but may reflect findings associated with a congenital abnormality such as Klippel-Feil syndrome (web neck, low-lying hairline, and limitation of neck motion) or a systemic disorder such as cancer. Torticollis, scoliosis, and facial asymmetry are common findings associated with congenital anomalies. A small, dysmorphic stature is found in patients with skeletal dysplasias, including achondroplasia, spondyloepiphyseal dysplasia, and other metabolic forms of dwarfism. Systemic disorders associated with CVJ abnormalities have a myriad of possible associated physical findings too numerous to include here. Careful attention to detail may help a practitioner reveal findings that unlock an associated diagnosis.

Neurological findings include myelopathy and cranial nerve palsies. Myelopathy presents as varying degrees of weakness or sensory disturbance in the upper or lower extremities. The myelopathy may mimic a "central cord syndrome" because of the preferential distribution of fibers subserving fine upper extremity motor movement within the corticospinal tract.[3] Motor myelopathy is attributed to repetitive trauma of the pyramidal tracts and chronic compression of the spinal cord at the cervicomedullary junction.[4] Bladder disturbance tends to parallel the motor myelopathy. Sensory myelopathy is most often manifested by symptoms associated with posterior column dysfunction. Cranial nerve and brain stem dysfunction produces a wide variety of findings. Sleep apnea, dysphagia, internuclear ophthalmoplegia, downbeat nystagmus, hearing loss,[3] and palatal/pharyngeal dysfunction are all common clinical manifestations of CVJ abnormalities. Abnormal cranial nerve signs may be attributed to trigeminal, glossopharyngeal, vagus, accessory, and hypoglossal nerve impingement.

Vascular insufficiency may produce symptoms or signs associated with basilar migraines, syncope, vertigo, intermittent hemiparesis, altered consciousness, or transient visual field loss. These findings may be associated with compression or occlusion of the vertebral artery, anterior spinal artery, or perforating arteries of the spinal cord. The vascular-related symptoms or signs may be provoked by craniocervical rotation or angulation, often as a result of occult occipitoatlantal or atlantoaxial instability.

## ◆ Management of Craniovertebral Junction Lesions

### Conservative Management

Only a minority of patients with CVJ abnormalities require surgery. Judicious patient selection and careful application of conservative measures may save a patient from inappropriate surgery and its attendant risks.[5] Algorithms that deal with CVJ problems may assist in the patient selection process (**Fig. 6–1**). Issues to

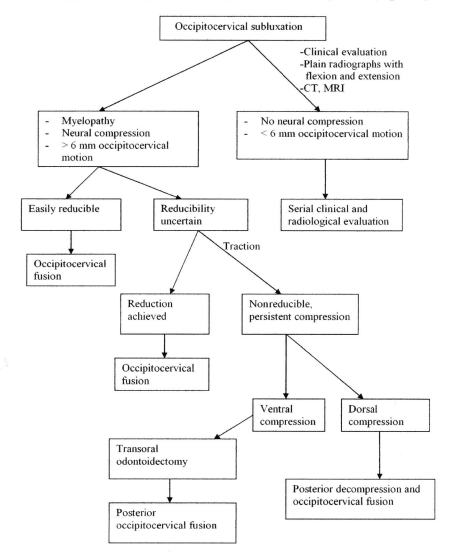

**Figure 6–1**  Algorithm for treatment of occipitocervical instability.

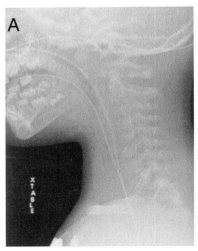
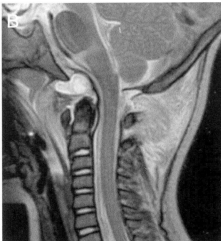
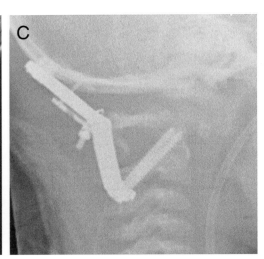

**Figure 6–2** A 22-month-old boy with atlanto-occipital dislocation (A–O dislocation), following a motor vehicle accident. **(A)** Preoperative lateral cervical spine film showing abnormal craniovertebral relationships consistent with AOD. **(B)** Preoperative midsagittal magnetic resonance imaging with short T1 inversion recovery sequence depicting significant posterior craniocervical soft tissue injury and craniocervical distraction. **(C)** Postoperative lateral cervical spine film showing occiput–C2 instrumentation with ABT loop (Medtronic Sofamor Danek, Memphis, TN), with C1–C2 transarticular screws with posterior occiput–C2 fusion.

be considered are the stability of the CVJ, the reducibility of the lesion, the presence or absence of neurovascular compression, the natural history of the disease, and the growth potential of the patient. Some patients with a stable CVJ and minimal or no neurological symptoms and potentially troublesome pathology (e.g., occipitalization of the atlas) may be managed safely with a soft cervical collar and seen in follow-up periodically. Others with a stable CVJ and a known benign natural history (e.g., an adolescent with Down syndrome[6]) may be reexamined only if symptoms occur. Obviously, clinical judgment must be exercised in each case.

Extremely young patients (such as newborns and those in the infant–toddler age group) with CVJ instability and pathology are generally managed with a custom-fitted external orthosis to provide protection and support until the patient is old enough to undergo operative management safely. As instrumentation and surgical techniques improve, however, it may be possible to provide operative stability in selected cases that obviously require fusion (**Figs. 6–2** and **6–3**). As time goes on, the strategies and techniques that dictate the management of this extremely challenging patient population will improve.

## Surgical Management and Decision Making

This section discusses various scenarios regarding the nature of a given CVJ lesion, its stability and reducibility, its natural history, and the patient's growth potential.

In general, if the major compressive lesion is from the anterior direction, an anterior approach (usually transoral) should be used, and dorsal fixation should be performed at the same time or as a staged procedure. Posterior compressive lesions may be dealt with by a strictly posterior approach. Lesions that have both anterior and posterior compression may be attacked from both directions and stabilized posteriorly.

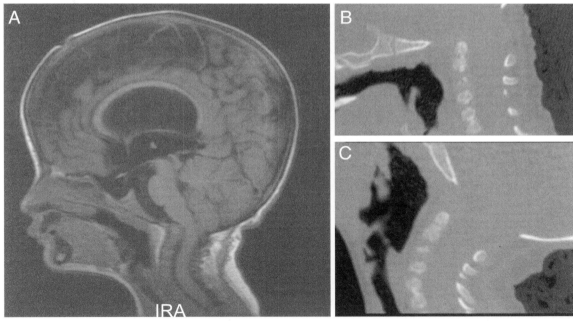

**Figure 6–3**    A 2$^{1}/_{2}$-year-old girl with severe congenital craniocervical instability. **(A)** Midsagittal T1-weighted magnetic resonance imaging scan showing significant craniocervical distortion and anterior brain stem compression. **(B)** Midsagittal two-dimensional computed tomographic (CT) reconstruction, with the patient in flexion, showing the severe craniocervical abnormalities. **(C)** Midsagittal two-dimensional CT reconstruction, with the patient in extension, showing reduction of deformity.

Unstable CVJ lesions must be stabilized at the time of surgery, usually from the posterior direction. Lesions that present with an initially stable CVJ may become unstable postoperatively following either or both removal of the mass and bony decompression and require fusion. Unless addressed at the initial surgery or shortly thereafter, this phenomenon will progress, especially in a vertical direction.

Irreducible lesions that require fusion should be fused in situ, whereas reducible lesions may be fused in their reduced position. Recent data from Larsson et al[7] have indicated that in situ posterior instrumentation and fusion alone in patients with rheumatoid arthritis can alleviate and potentially improve anterior compressive lesions and symptoms. How this information may apply to pediatric patients with similar inflammatory pathology is unknown.

Growth considerations in children with CVJ pathology are a major factor, both from the standpoint of obtaining proper fixation and fusion and for the potential for postoperative spinal deformity or juxtafusion pathology. Our 10-year experience with rigid screw fixation constructs in more than 50 pediatric patients ages 18 months to 16 years supports the notion that growth arrest occurs at the affected level after successful fusion and that spinal deformity below the fusion does not occur. Therefore, we believe that posterior occipitocervical screw fixation and fusion may be routinely performed down to ~2 to 3 years of age. Other authors have described instrumentation, such as the inside-out technique,[8] which is also appropriate for very young patients, although several cervical motion segments must be sacrificed to obtain proper fixation. Obviously, the anatomical suitability of younger patients must be evaluated on a case-by-case basis.

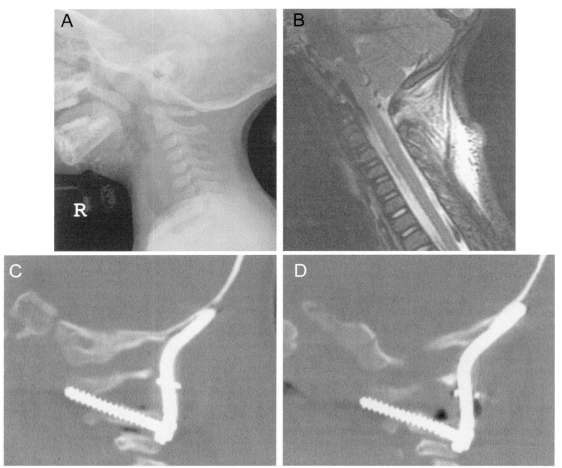

**Figure 6–4**    A 4-year-old boy with atlanto-occipital dislocation. **(A)** Preoperative plain lateral cervical spine film. **(B)** Preoperative midsagittal magnetic resonance imaging with short T1 inversion recovery sequence showing severe posterior soft tissue injury. **(C)** Right and **(D)** left parasagittal two-dimensional computed tomographic reconstruction of craniocervical instrumentation, using ABT plate (Medtronic Sofamor Danek, Minneapolis, MN), respectively.

Size-for-age constraints may also be encountered in patients with CVJ pathology. For example, a 12-year-old patient with spondyloepiphyseal dysplasia may have a vertebral column the size of a normal 5-year-old child. Therefore, the surgeon must be comfortable working with smaller patients and the distorted anatomy that may be encountered (**Fig. 6–4**).

## ◆ Surgical Approaches

Multiple surgical approaches to the CVJ have been described over the years. These approaches can be broken down into anterior, anterolateral, and posterior/posterolateral. To decide whether a given approach is appropriate for a given lesion, one must be familiar with all of the potential approaches for that lesion and their accompanying risks and benefits. In general, the shortest distance from the lesion to the skin defines the trajectory of the approach, or one very close to it.

Anterior approaches include transoral,[9-14] transoral-extended maxillotomy,[15-20] transoral-translabiomandibular,[21] and transfacial.[22-24] The basic transoral approach provides exposure from the bottom portion of the clivus to the bottom of C2. If one divides the hard palate, exposure to the upper part of the clivus is obtained. Each variation of the transoral approach listed here provides exposure to various anatomical regions, which may extend from the anterior cranial fossa superiorly to the outer portions of the maxilla laterally, depending on the variation chosen.

The CVJ can be exposed directly from an anterolateral direction via a far lateral suboccipital approach,[25-27] a retropharyngeal approach,[28-30] or a mandibular swing-transcervical approach.[31] Anterolateral skull base approaches that are commonly extended down to the CVJ include the infratemporal fossa[32-34] and transpetrosal exposures.[35,36] Similarly, anterolateral approaches to the cervical spine may be extended up to the CVJ.[26,37]

Posterior and posterolateral exposures of the CVJ include the traditional midline posterior approach, with or without a suboccipital craniotomy/craniectomy, the retrosigmoid approach,[38] and posterolateral approaches to the cervical spine.[26,37,39,40] The midline posterior approach is the most common approach used to the CVJ because most of the fusion and instrumentation techniques available rely on dorsal points of fixation.

## ◆ Implants

If a pathological process at the CVJ produces instability at the occipitoatlantal or atlantoaxial joints, or if surgical resection of a lesion produces instability at those levels, instrumentation and fusion are necessary to provide long-term protection of the neural elements and prevent further spinal deformity. Depending on which level requires stabilization, a variety of instrumentation and fusion techniques are available.

For occipitoatlantal instability, posterior occipitocervical instrumentation from the occiput to C2 level is typically performed. One of the traditional constructs that is still very popular today includes a contoured loop with sublaminar and occipital wire (or cable) fixation, with or without an external halo orthosis.[11,41] Recent advances in screw fixation techniques, however, have allowed surgeons to couple C1–C2 transarticular or C2 pedicle screws to rigid loops, plates, or rod–plate constructs that span the occipitocervical region, yielding very high rates of fusion without the need for an external orthosis. Brockmeyer and Apfelbaum,[42] Pait et al,[8] Schultz et al,[43] and Vale et al[44] have all described different methods of coupling C1–C2 transarticular or pedicle screws into occipitocervical constructs. The type of occipital fixation used varies from author to author and includes direct screw placement[42,44] and transosseous couplers.[8] A recent publication describes considerable success with anchoring occipital-cervical U-loops or plates with direct screw fixation.[45] In that article, 25 patients underwent occipitocervical fusion with that technique, 24 without halos or external orthoses, with 100% successful fusion. Three complications occurred, all successfully treated infections.

A new occipitocervical plate, specifically designed for use in pediatric patients, has been developed. Manufactured by Medtronic Sofamor Danek (Minneapolis, MN), it is known as the Avery–Brockmeyer–Thiokol (ABT) plate. The ABT plate is manufactured in several different sizes corresponding to different ages of patients. Preliminary experience with the device has been encouraging; fusion occurred in all 15 patients in which it has been implanted. The implantation of the ABT plate is described later in this chapter.

## ◆ Bone Graft Materials

Posterior iliac crest autograft is the preferred substrate for bone graft material in pediatric occipitocervical fusions. Iliac crest is readily available, can be harvested with a minimum of morbidity, and is highly adaptable to the unique location in which it is placed. Other authors have described using split-thickness occipital bone for posterior occipitocervical fusions, but this is rarely practical in the thin bone of a child. The only other viable alternative is to use rib graft, which is enthusiastically supported by this author in cases where iliac crest graft is not available (e.g., after multiple fusion attempts) or when the anticipated quality of the iliac crest bone is poor (e.g., in very young children or non-weight-bearing older children such as those with spina bifida).

In the author's experience and opinion, under no circumstance should either structural or morcellized allograft be used as a posterior onlay graft for occipitocervical fusions. The author has revised three failed occipitocervical fusions where the failure has been directly attributable to the use of allograft. In contrast, in the author's personal series, no occipitocervical fusion failures have occurred when autograft has been used.

## ◆ External Orthoses

Typically, after a rigid occipitocervical screw fixation and fusion, a patient is placed either in a soft cervical collar for comfort or in a hard cervical collar if some restriction in craniovertebral motion is desirable (e.g., in Down syndrome patients who may not understand they must have activity limitations). Given their relatively high rate of complications,[5,46,47] every effort is made to avoid placing the patient in a halo postoperatively; however, occasionally circumstances make an external orthosis desirable. These circumstances include cases where bone quality is poor and screw purchase may be compromised (e.g., osteomyelitis or tumor) or congenital bony anomalies prevent adequate screw placement. As already described, out of 25 patients who underwent occipitocervical fusion at our institution, only one required a halo for inadequate screw purchase caused by congenital vertebral anomalies. The author believes that the routine use of halo orthoses following occipitocervical fusion is not necessary in the era of advanced internal fixation.[45]

## ◆ Postoperative Follow-up

At our institution, each patient is followed carefully with a specific imaging protocol following occipitocervical fusion. Plain lateral cervical spine films are obtained at 1, 2, and 3 months postsurgery to document the integrity of the hardware while bony fusion is taking place. At 4 months postsurgery, the patient undergoes a thin-cut CT scan from occiput to C3 with two-dimensional reconstructions of the parasagittal and coronal planes to determine whether the arthrodesis has taken. A continuous bony bridge between the occiput and the posterior elements of C2 must be seen to state that the patient has fused successfully. If the fusion has not taken and the imaging suggests that it eventually will, the CT scan is repeated at approximately 2- to 3-month intervals. Fusions that have obviously failed are revised in a timely manner with autologous iliac crest bone graft.

Patients are followed with yearly plain lateral cervical spine films to assess overall spinal alignment, growth, and the presence of juxtafusion pathology.

## ◆ An Advanced Technique for Occipitocervical Fusion

For purposes of teaching occipitocervical instrumentation, this chapter focuses on the technique of C1–C2 transarticular screw fixation coupled to an occipitocervical plate. For details regarding the placement of C1–C2 transarticular screws in children, please refer to Chapter 5, Advanced Atlantoaxial Surgery in Children.

After induction of general endotracheal anesthesia, the patient is placed into Mayfield pin headholders and then turned into the prone position. Intraoperative fluoroscopy is used to assist placement of the patient's CVJ into appropriate anatomical alignment. Because the initial goal is to place C1–C2 transarticular or pedicle screws, a slightly flexed, "military" neck position is preferred. During final placement of the occipitocervical plate, the patient's neck is placed back into a more neutral position.

A midline occipitocervical incision is made from the inion to C4, and the paraspinous musculature is stripped to the side. Headless C1–C2 transarticular screws (Medtronic Sofamor Danek, Minneapolis, MN) are placed bilaterally using the techniques described in Chapter 5. The distance between the transarticular screws becomes the distance that dictates the size of the ABT occipital-cervical plate (Medtronic Sofamor Danek) (**Fig. 6–5**). The plate holes are then placed over the headless screws, and the screw heads are applied and tightened

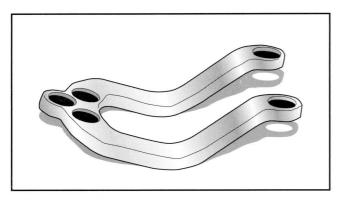

**Figure 6–5**    Side view of ABT plate (Medtronic Sofamor Danek, Memphis, TN).

(**Figs. 6–6, 6–7,** and **6–8**). It may be necessary to drill or rongeur away bone to assure that the plate lies flat against the lamina of C2. Screws measuring 10 mm length by 4 mm width outer diameter (OD) are placed into the midline occipital keel and adjacent occipital bone using standard drilling and tapping techniques (**Figs. 6–9** and **6–10**).

A posterior iliac crest bone graft is harvested and shaped to fit between the plate arms laterally and the occipital–C2 complex. The bone surfaces meant to be in contact with one another (i.e., the occiput and upper part of the graft; C2 and the lower part of the graft) are decorticated with a high-speed drill. The graft is held in place with a multistranded titanium cable through its midsection and a 12 mm length by 4 mm width OD screw in its upper portion (**Fig. 6–11**). Ten cubic centimeters of Grafton Demineralized Bone Matrix (Osteotech, Eatontown, NJ) is placed around the fusion construct. The wound is then closed in layers.

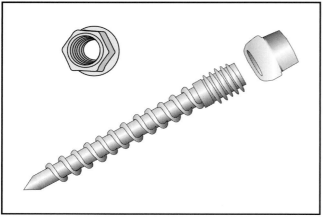

**Figure 6–6**    Headless screw with nut used with ABT plate (Medtronic Sofamor Danek, Memphis, TN).

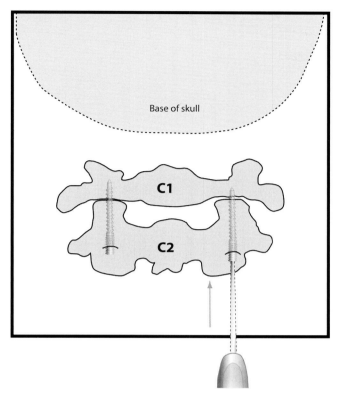

**Figure 6–7**   Illustration demonstrating placement of C1–C2 headless screws.

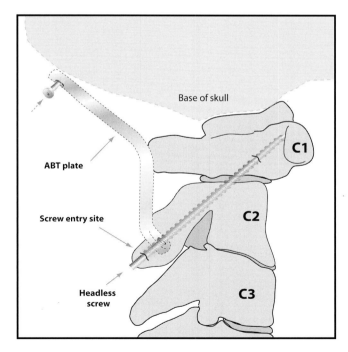

**Figure 6–8**   Screw trajectory seen in lateral fluoroscopic view.

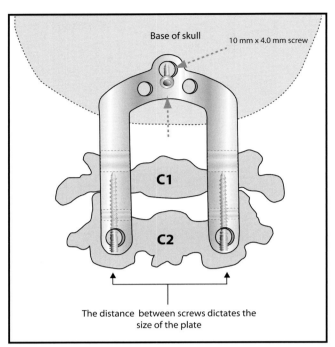

**Figure 6–9**    Final placement of ABT plate (Medtronic Sofamor Danek,  Memphis, TN) and headless screws.

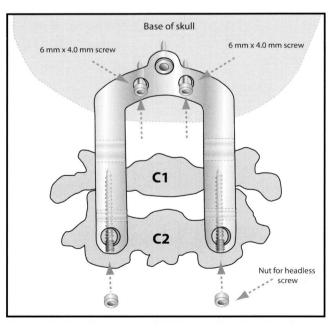

**Figure 6–10**    Placement of ABT plate (Medtronic Sofamor Danek, Memphis, TN) and nut on headless screws (countertorque tightener required).

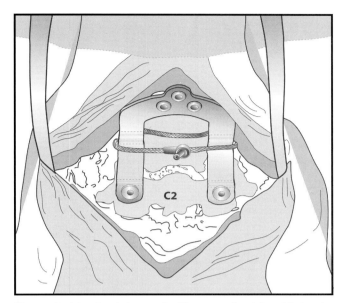

**Figure 6–11**   Occipitocervical bone graft with cable in place.

## References

1. Menezes A. Embryology, development, and classification of the craniovertebral junction. In: Dickman C, Spetzler R, Sonntag V, eds. Surgery of the Craniovertebral Junction. New York: Thieme; 1998:3–12

2. Menezes A. Craniovertebral anomalies and syringomyelia. In: Choux M, Rocco CD, Hockley A, Walker M, eds. Pediatric Neurosurgery. London: Harcourt Brace; 1999:151–184

3. Levi AD, Tator CH, Bunge RP. Clinical syndromes associated with disproportionate weakness of the upper versus the lower extremities after cervical spinal cord injury. Neurosurgery 1996;38:179–183

4. Dickman C, Hadley M, Pappas C. Cruciate paralysis: a clinical and radiographic analysis of injuries to the cervicomedullary junction. J Neurosurg 1990;73: 850–858

5. Rockswold GL, Bergman TA, Ford SE. Halo immobilization and surgical fusion: relative indications and effectiveness in the treatment of 140 cervical spine injuries. J Trauma 1990;30:893–898

6. Brockmeyer D. Down syndrome and craniovertebral instability: topic review and treatment recommendations. Pediatr Neurosurg 1999;31:71–77

7. Larsson E, Holtas S, Zygmunt S. Pre- and postoperative MR imaging of the craniocervical junction in rheumatoid arthritis. AJR Am J Roentgenol 1989;152: 561–566

8. Pait T, Al-Mefty O, Boop F, Arnautovic K, Rahman S, Ceola W. Inside–outside technique for posterior occipitocervical spine instrumentation and stabilization: preliminary results. J Neurosurg 1999;90:1–7

9. Crockard H, Pozo J, Ransford A, et al. Transoral decompression and posterior fusion for rheumatoid atlanto-axial subluxation. J Bone Joint Surg Br 1986;68:350–356

10. Menezes A, VanGilder J. Transoral-transpharyngeal approach to the anterior craniocervical junction: ten-year experience with 72 patients. J Neurosurg 1988;69:895–903

11. Menezes A, VanGilder J, Graf C, et al. Craniocervical abnormalities: a comprehensive surgical approach. J Neurosurg 1980;53:444–455

12. Mullan S, Naunton R, Hekmat-Panah J, et al. The use of an anterior approach to ventrally placed tumors in the foramen magnum and vertebral column. J Neurosurg 1966;24:536–543

13. Scoville W, Sherman I. Platybasia: report of ten cases with comments of familial tendency, a special diagnostic sign, and the end results of operation. Ann Surg 1951;133:496–502

14. Spetzler RF, Selman WR, Nash CL Jr, et al. Transoral microsurgical odontoid resection and spinal cord monitoring. Spine 1979;4:506–510

15. Bowles A, Suen J, Al-Mefty O. Unilateral open-door maxillotomy for lesions of the clivus. Skull Base Surg 1994;4:26

16. Crockard H, Johnston F. Development of transoral approaches to lesions of the skull base and craniovertebral junction. Neurosurg Quart 1993;3:61–82

17. Crockard H, Sen C. The transoral approach for the management of intradural lesions at the craniovertebral junction: review of 7 cases. Neurosurgery 1991;28:88–98

18. Harkey H, Crockard H, Stevens J, Smith R, Ransford A. The operative management of basilar impression in osteogenesis imperfecta. Neurosurgery 1990;27:782–786

19. Harkey H, Crockard H. Transoral-extended maxillotomy. In: Dickman C, Spetzler R, Sonntag V, eds. Surgery of the Craniovertebral Junction. New York: Thieme; 1998:371–381

20. James D, Crockard H. Surgical access to the base of skull and upper cervical spine by extended maxillotomy. Neurosurgery 1991;29:411–416

21. Janecka I. Transoral-translabiomandibular approach to the craniovertebral junction. In: Dickman C, Spetzler R, Sonntag V, eds. Surgery of the Craniovertebral Junction. New York: Thieme; 1998:383–393

22. Beals S, Joganic E. Transfacial exposure of anterior cranial fossa and clival tumors. BNI Q 1992;8:2–18

23. Beals S, Joganic E. Transfacial approaches to the craniovertebral junction. In: Dickman C, Spetzler R, Sonntag V, eds. Surgery of the Craniovertebral Junction. New York: Thieme; 1998:395–418

24. Sandor GK, Charles DA, Lawson VG, et al. Transoral approach to the nasopharynx and clivus using the Le Fort I osteotomy with midpalatal split. Int J Oral Maxillofac Surg 1990;19:352–355

25. Heros R. Lateral suboccipital approach for vertebral and vertebrobasilar artery lesions. J Neurosurg 1986;64:559–562

26. Sen C, Sekhar L. An extreme lateral approach to intradural lesions of the cervical spine and foramen magnum. Neurosurgery 1990;27:197–204

27. Spetzler R, Grahm T. The far-lateral approach to the inferior clivus and the upper cervical region: technical note. BNI Q 1990;6:35–38

28. Vardiman A, Dickman C, Sonntag V. Modified anterolateral retropharyngeal approach to the craniovertebral junction. In: Dickman C, Spetzler R, Sonntag V, eds. Surgery of the Craniovertebral Junction. New York: Thieme; 1998:419–431

29. Riley L. Surgical approaches to the anterior structures of the cervical spine. Clin Orthop 1973;91:16–20

30. McAfee P, Bohlman H, Riley L, et al. The anterior retropharyngeal approach to the upper part of the cervical spine. J Bone Joint Surg 1987;69:1371–1383

31. Ammirati M, Ma J, Cheatham M, Mei Z, Bloch J, Becker D. The mandibular swing-transcervical approach to the skull base: anatomical study: technical note. J Neurosurg 1993;78:673–681

32. Sen C, Sekhar L. The subtemporal and preauricular infratemporal approach to intradural structures ventral to the brain stem. J Neurosurg 1990;73:345–354

33. Fisch U, Pillsbury H. Infratemporal fossa approach to lesions in the temporal bone and base of the skull. Arch Otolaryngol 1979;105:99–107

34. Bertalanffy H, Seeger W. The dorsolateral, suboccipital, transcondylar approach to the lower clivus and anterior portion of the craniocervical junction. Neurosurgery 1991;29:815–821

35. Al-Mefty O, Fox J, Smith R. Petrosal approach for petroclival meningiomas. Neurosurgery 1988;22:510–517

36. Spetzler R, Caspit C, Pappas C. The combined supra- and infratentorial approach for lesions of the petrous and clival regions: experience with 46 cases. J Neurosurg 1992;76:588–599

37. Shucart W, Kleriga E. A lateral approach to the upper cervical spine. Neurosurgery 1980;6:278–281

38. Rhoton A. Suboccipital and retrosigmoid approaches to the craniovertebral junction. In: Dickman C, Spetzler R, Sonntag V, eds. Surgery of the Craniovertebral Junction. New York: Thieme; 1998:659–681

39. Verbiest H. A lateral approach to the cervical spine: technique and indications. J Neurosurg 1968;28:191–203

40. Whitesides T, Kelly R. Lateral approach to the upper cervical spine for anterior fusion. South Med J 1966;59:879–883

41. Menezes A, VanGilder J. Anomalies of the craniovertebral junction. In: Youmans J, ed. Neurological Surgery. Philadelphia: WB Saunders; 1990:1359–1420

42. Brockmeyer DL, Apfelbaum RI. A new occipitocervical fusion construct in pediatric patients with occipitocervical instability. J Neurosurg 1999;90:271–275

43. Schultz KD Jr, Petronio J, Haid RW, et al. Pediatric occipitocervical arthrodesis: a review of current options and early evaluation of rigid internal fixation techniques. Pediatr Neurosurg 2000;33:169–181

44. Vale F, Oliver M, Cahill DW. Rigid occipitocervical fusion. J Neurosurg 1999;91:144–150

45. Gluf WM, Brockmeyer DL. Atlantoaxial transarticular screw fixation: a review of surgical indications, fusion rate, complications, and lessons learned in 67 pediatric patients. J Neurosurg Spine 2005;2:164–169

46. Lennarson PJ, Mostafavi H, Traynelis VC, Walters BC. Management of type II dens fractures: a case-control study. Spine 2000;25:1234–1237

47. Thompson RC Jr, Meyer TJ. Posterior surgical stabilization for atlantoaxial subluxation in rheumatoid arthritis. Spine 1985;10:597–601

# 7

# Advanced Surgery for the Subaxial Cervical Spine in Children

**Douglas L. Brockmeyer**

Management of disorders in the subaxial cervical spine in children is a complex and challenging endeavor. The main challenge faced by pediatric spine surgeons is the broad range of patient ages they must manage and the various physiologies they represent. For example, on one end of the age spectrum, the pediatric spine surgeon sees teenagers with adult-type cervical spine physiology and pathology. Therefore, the surgeon must be knowledgeable about adult-type treatment principles regarding the cervical spine. On the other hand, complex, fascinating, and sometimes bewildering conditions occur at the other end of the age spectrum in newborn children or toddlers. These conditions may defy conventional management strategies. For patients between these extremes, surgeons must use their best judgment regarding the most appropriate treatment for a particular patient, borrowing heavily from their training in adult spine surgery.

This chapter synthesizes several important principles regarding advanced subaxial cervical spine surgery in children. It will begin by reviewing the clinical presentation of patients with these disorders and then will provide a detailed examination of their surgical and nonsurgical management. Finally, it will present several of the author's preferred techniques for managing both straightforward and challenging cases of the pediatric cervical spine.

## ◆ Clinical Findings

The clinical presentation of cervical spine disorders in children is highly variable. Pain, weakness, sensory change, autonomic disturbance, or spine deformity may exist alone or in combination as the presenting complaints. Cervical spine pain is the most common presenting symptom and is almost universally found in the setting of a traumatic injury. Posttraumatic pain may be isolated to the neck area or may be radicular. Cervical spine pain, especially pain on motion, that lingers after a traumatic injury is abnormal and should be investigated. Like pain, weakness and sensory change may follow a radicular pattern, but they can also be part of a myelopathic syndrome involving a certain vertebral level. Autonomic disturbances, including bowel and bladder changes, may also occur but are uncommon. Urinary incontinence may be an early finding in a history suggestive of autonomic instability. Cervical spine and craniovertebral deformity, including torticollis or scoliosis, may be recognized at birth or noticed later in life. In addition, some congenital cervical spine deformities may be diagnosed as an incidental finding on a routine chest radiograph.

The physical examination of a known or suspected cervical spine disorder should proceed in a stepwise manner. General findings may be specific to a certain congenital vertebral syndrome or may suggest other syndromes associated with congenital vertebral anomalies. For instance, a low-lying hairline or web-neck deformity may suggest Klippel-Feil syndrome. Features consistent with Down syndrome are readily apparent. Abnormalities of the ears or palate may be associated with Goldenhar's syndrome, and café au lait spots are indicative of neurofibromatosis type 1.

Examination of the extremities should be performed next. Generalized ligamentous laxity may suggest Ehlers-Danlos syndrome or Larsen's syndrome. Foot deformities, such as high arches or cavus abnormalities, are associated with Friedreich's ataxia. The association of foot and spine deformities strongly suggests spinal dysraphism or a generalized neuromuscular disorder.

Physical examination of the cervical spine is centered on the assessment of pain and mobility. Pain in the form of paravertebral muscle spasm is commonly found in posttraumatic injuries. Localized "trigger points" in the myofascial planes usually indicate a soft tissue injury and do not necessarily indicate cervical instability is present. Patients with significant posttraumatic instability have a deep, unrelenting pain in their cervical spine and are hesitant to move their neck. Given that, it is important to note how much motion is present in the cardinal planes of motion (flexion, extension, lateral bending, rotation) in each patient. The presence of Lhermitte's-type symptoms on flexion or extension should also be noted. Scoliosis of the cervical spine should be described by the curve's apex and location.

A complete neurological examination should be performed as well. Particular emphasis should be placed on the cranial nerve examination, sensorimotor testing, and deep tendon and plantar reflexes. These tests form the foundation for neurological localization in spinal cord disease. Any decrease in muscle bulk or change in muscle tone should also be sought and may aid in localizing value. The patient's gait and station may provide subtle clues for the presence of lower extremity or truncal weakness.

## ◆ Management of Subaxial Cervical Spine Lesions

### Conservative Management

Conservative management of subaxial cervical spine abnormalities in children is used when the patient fails to meet criteria required for operative intervention. Such circumstances include traumatic injuries where the bony and ligamentous damage is not severe enough to result in progressive deformity or neurological insult, or very young patients where a congenital abnormality is present but not progressively deteriorating (**Fig. 7–1**). The decision not to proceed with surgery is sometimes harder to make than the decision to proceed to the operating room. If the decision is not to operate, most patients are kept in a standard hard cervical collar and followed carefully with appropriate serial radiographs. The radiographic gold standard for determining whether a cervical spine is stable is plain spine x-rays with flexion and extension views. These views must be obtained after the patient's posttraumatic paravertebral spasm has subsided, usually 2 to 3 weeks after the injury. Very young patients with congenital subaxial cervical spine abnormalities may require a custom cervical collar or external orthosis to provide support and stability while the child is

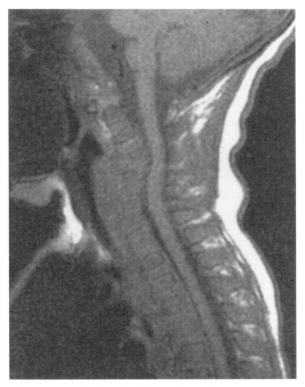

**Figure 7–1**   Midsagittal T1-weighted magnetic resonance imaging scan, depicting a congenitally narrow spinal canal in a 10-month-old boy. Note severe congenital narrowing from C3 down to C5.

growing. Again, appropriate serial radiographs are required to determine whether the child's spine and spinal cord remain out of danger.

## Surgical Management and Decision Making

The decision to operate on a child with a cervical spine lesion below C2 is based on several factors. Evidence of cervical spine instability, neurological deficit caused by compressive lesion, and progressive deformity are the main criteria on which the decision is based. Radiographic evidence of cervical spine instability is by no means absolute, but the following findings are helpful guidelines: vertebral body angulation greater than 15 degrees, vertebral body subluxation greater than 5 mm, or unilateral or bilateral locked facets. Pang (unpublished data) has shown evidence that a kyphotic angulation of greater than 7 degrees represents significant ligamentous injury and predisposes the juvenile cervical spine to further kyphosis and instability.

Neurological deficits caused by unstable cervical spine injuries should lead to surgical stabilization; however, it can sometimes be difficult to determine whether a cervical spine lesion is unstable. For example, many spinal cord deficits caused by the so-called spinal cord injury without radiographic abnormality (SCIWORA)–type injury are clearly not caused by an unstable lesion. In these cases, radiographic studies are normal, and the patient is usually treated in a conservative fashion, perhaps even in a hard cervical spine collar for 1 to 3 months. On the other hand, some cervical spinal cord injuries caused by SCI-WORA-type mechanisms have evidence of ligamentous injury on magnetic resonance imaging (MRI) and normal flexion and extension cervical spine films. Such patients should be followed carefully with serial cervical spine flexion and extension films to rule out late instability. We have seen several patients over the years develop late instability in these circumstances. As already noted, identifying patients with greater than 7 degrees of kyphotic angulation on a plain lateral cervical spine x-ray can provide a helpful guideline for managing children with incipient instability. Those patients are at high risk of developing further angulation and ultimately might require surgical stabilization.

Other circumstances that call for careful decision making are injuries in which major supportive structures of the spine, such as the transverse ligament of C2 or subaxial disk space, are completely destroyed by a penetrating injury. Gunshot wounds and knife injuries can produce these lesions. Although static films and MRI scans may show good anatomical continuity, the known effects of missing these important structures should compel the surgeon to either stabilize the patient surgically or follow the patient very carefully with serial dynamic x-rays.

Compressive mass lesions causing neurological deficits should be resected, although the resection may leave the cervical spine unstable. The decision as to whether the spine should be stabilized at the time of surgery may be simple or somewhat complicated. It is usually based on whether significant portions of the anterior or posterior column are resected, or on whether stabilizing the spine would prevent a progressive deformity in the future. Lesions that call for complete removal of a vertebral body, disk space, or bilateral facet complex should probably be fused at the time of the initial surgery. Consideration should also be given to whether the patient may require postoperative radiation or

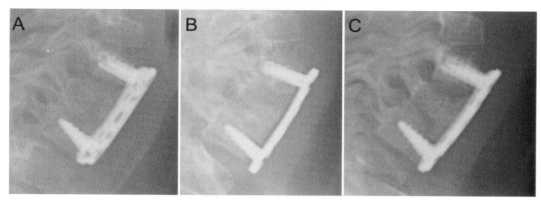

**Figure 7–2**  A 6-year-old boy with a large C6 eosinophilic granuloma. He underwent an anterior cervical C6 corpectomy and fusion with anterior plating using an ABC plate (Aesculap, Inc., Center Valley, PA). He also underwent chemotherapy for eosinophilic granulomas in other organ systems. **(A)** Plain lateral cervical spine film taken immediately after surgery. **(B)** Plain lateral cervical spine film taken 4 months after surgery showing lack of bony arthrodesis from C4 to C6. **(C)** Plain lateral cervical spine film taken 10 months after surgery showing incomplete, but adequate, bony arthrodesis from C4 to C6.

chemotherapy, which may have an influence on the stability of the cervical spine. Patients who undergo fusion and then radiation or chemotherapy may require extra time to fuse, perhaps as long as 6 months or a year. As long as the internal hardware remains intact and the fusion mass does not show evidence of resorption, it is safe to observe the patient with serial x-rays (**Fig. 7–2**).

Prevention of cervical spine deformity and maintenance of normal cervical spine alignment are very important. It is better to have a normally aligned fused cervical spine than a nonfused spine with the potential for malalignment. Reconstructing the cervical spine after a multilevel resection can be demanding, and careful attention must be paid to achieving as close to normal alignment as possible (**Figs. 7–3** and **7–4**).

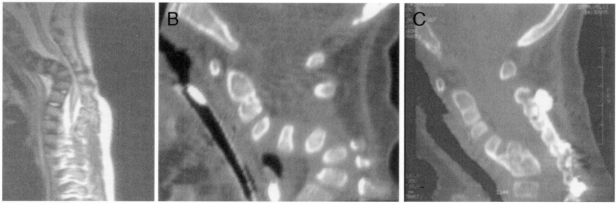

**Figure 7–3**  A 3-year-old girl with arthrogryposis and congenital cervical swan neck deformity. **(A)** T2-weighted midsagittal magnetic resonance imaging showing lower cervical kyphotic abnormality with severe cord compression. **(B)** Midsagittal two-dimensional computed tomographic (CT) reconstruction showing severe lower cervical kyphotic abnormality with canal narrowing. **(C)** Midsagittal two-dimensional CT reconstruction. One year after a combined anterior and posterior fusion, the film shows a solid bony arthrodesis in the posterior and anterior columns.

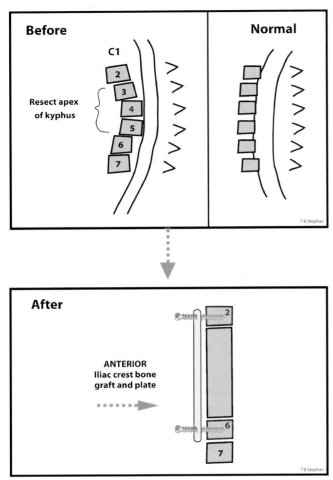

**Figure 7–4**   Management of multilevel cervical spondylolysis with kyphosis.

## ◆ Surgical Approaches

### Anterior Cervical Approach

The traditional anterior cervical approach is highly versatile and can be adapted for use in patients of any age. The surgical exposure provides visualization of at least three vertebral body segments and two disk spaces at a time. The incision may be moved superior or inferior in the neck to reach from the body of C2 down to at least T1. Depending on the body habitus of the patient, T2 or T3 can be reached as well. Great care must be taken to avoid injury to the carotid artery, trachea, and esophagus. Transient recurrent laryngeal nerve palsies occur occasionally but almost always recover on their own. No studies have looked at the incidence of recurrent laryngeal nerve palsies in children, but in the author's experience, they are uncommon and self-limited. Keeping the incision in a skin crease minimizes scarring and makes for a pleasing cosmetic result. Implanting anterior cervical arthrodeses and instrumentation is a straightforward matter using this approach.

## Cervical Anterolateral Approach

The cervical anterolateral approach, perhaps better known as the retropharyngeal approach, has been well described in the literature. It has been described for use mostly in adults, and is used only occasionally in children. It is appropriate for resection of lesions lateral and high in the cervical spine that cannot be accessed by a strictly anterior or posterior approach or that may need a combined approach. Details of the approach have been described by McAfee et al[1] and Vardiman et al.[2]

## Posterior Midline Approach

The posterior midline approach to the cervical spine is commonly performed and highly adaptable. With proper attention to bony removal and handling of the muscle, lesions extending to the anterolateral portion of the spinal canal can be accessed and resected. Postresection instrumentation and fusion to provide stabilization from the posterior direction are usually anchored by lateral mass or pedicle screws joined by rods or plates (**Fig. 7–5**). Other types of

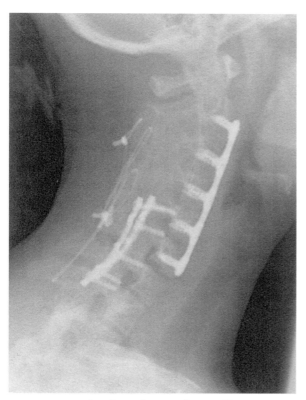

**Figure 7–5**  Plain lateral cervical spine film in a 12-year-old girl with neurofibromatosis, with combined anterior and posterior fusion constructs.

bone-and-wire (or cable) constructs have been described and are used extensively. The posterior approach does cause significantly more postoperative discomfort than the anterior approach because of paravertebral muscle spasm, and, for that reason, the author believes it should not be used routinely but rather when the pathology mandates an approach from a posterior direction.

## ◆ Implants

### Anterior Plates

Anterior cervical plate and screw designs, first introduced in the mid-1980s by Wolfhard Caspar et al,[3] have undergone considerable evolution. The initial plates were rigid and relied on bicortical screw purchase of the vertebral bodies to achieve much of their strength. Later anterior cervical plate designs introduced features such as locking mechanisms to prevent screw backout, self-tapping screws, and dynamic plate movement to prevent stress shielding. These concepts and designs will not be reviewed in detail here except to illustrate important points regarding placement of anterior cervical plates in children.

Placing anterior cervical plates in children is unique because the pediatric cervical spine is different anatomically from the adult cervical spine. A smaller vertebral body radius of curvature, smaller disk space height, smaller vertebral body height, and an increased amount of cartilaginous end plate all contribute to a surgical environment that not only does not accept adult-sized surgical implants but also is particularly unyielding to technical error. For instance, once the disk space and cartilaginous end plate have been resected in preparation for placement of an interbody graft, there is not much vertebral body height left in which to place a screw. Errors in screw hole placement may lead to the screw traversing into the adjacent disk space or the inability to redrill a hole if the proper trajectory is not taken. In essence, screw hole placement in a small pediatric vertebral body is critical and must be performed correctly the first time.

Anterior cervical plates can be divided into two large categories: rigid or dynamic systems. A brief look at each may help the surgeon choose which type of system to use.

### Rigid Anterior Cervical Plates

Rigid anterior cervical plate systems were originally designed for the adult population and have been available for more than a decade. During the past several years, new versions of adult-type plating systems have been designed to accommodate the pediatric population. The Short Stature Anterior Cervical Spine Locking Plate (Synthes, Inc., West Chester, PA) and the Zephyr plate (Medtronic Sofamor Danek, Memphis, TN) are the best examples of plates specifically designed for use in children as young as approximately 5 years. They are also useful for providing rigid internal stabilization in adults of short stature. The advantages of pediatric-sized anterior cervical plates over adult-sized plates include smaller overall dimensions, lower profiles, and a reduced radius of curvature. The Synthes and Sofamor Danek systems also include self-tapping screws, locking screw mechanisms, and prebent lordotic shapes. The disadvantages of these systems include their rigid design, which may contribute to stress shielding and fusion failure in certain patients, and the inability to tap the screw hole before a screw is placed, which may lead to pressure necrosis in the bone surrounding the screw and, ultimately, screw failure or breakage. The author has successfully used the Zephyr plate for anterior cervical corpectomies or diskectomies in patients as young as 3 years old. For patients 5 years of age or older, the author prefers a dynamic anterior cervical plate construct.

## Dynamic Anterior Cervical Plates

Dynamic anterior cervical plate systems are a new addition to the cervical spine surgical armamentarium. Dynamic anterior cervical plates work by allowing for graft subsidence and load sharing between the graft and the plate. Over time, they have proven to be very successful in contributing to cervical stabilization and fusion. A growing body of literature suggests that for almost every surgical indication, dynamic plates are at least as good as, and perhaps superior to, rigid plates in providing an environment in which a surgical fusion can take place.[4,5] The ABC plate (Aesculap, Inc., Center Valley, PA) is currently one of the most highly evolved of the dynamic plate systems and offers several features that are attractive to the pediatric spine surgeon (**Fig. 7–6**). These include small

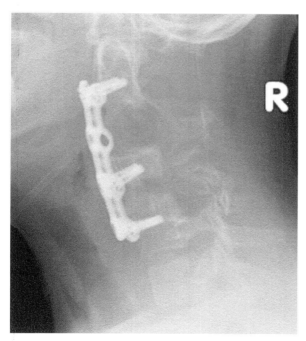

**Figure 7–6**    Plain lateral cervical spine film in a 14-year-old girl with Klippel-Feil deformity and severe multilevel cervical instability. Note the presence of the ABC plate from C2 down to C6.

dimensions, low profiles, and a reduced radius of curvature. The only disadvantage to this system is that it is not adaptable to small patients, such as those under 5 years of age. The Zephyr plate (Medtronic Sofamor Danek) is probably a better choice in that circumstance. Although there are currently no biomechanical or clinical data examining the subject of dynamic plates in the pediatric population, it seems reasonable to expect that the same success seen in the adult population with dynamic plates will translate to children as well. So far, the author's 5-year experience with dynamic plates in children has yielded encouraging results.

## Posterior Plate and Rod Systems

An alternate approach for pediatric subaxial cervical spine stabilization, which may be used alone or in combination with an anterior plate, involves posterior plate and rod systems. Typical indications for placing such systems include (1) providing stability in an unstable spine, (2) maintaining alignment to allow fusion to occur, (3) preventing further progression of deformity, and (4) alleviating pain.

Posterior plate and rod systems are typically anchored by screws placed either in the pedicle or in the pars interarticularis. To achieve fixation, the screws can be passed directly through a solid plate at two or more levels using a method popularized by Roy-Camille in the 1980s,[6] or the screws can be joined with a top-loading rod system. One example of the plate design is the Small Notched Plate (Synthes USA, Paoli, PA). Examples of the top-loading rod systems include Vertex (Medtronic Sofamor Danek, Memphis, TN), Summit (DePuy/Acromed, Cleveland, OH), and Starlock (Synthes USA, Paoli, PA). Liu and Das[7] in 2001 provided a detailed review of the indications and techniques for these systems in adults, but this subject has not been examined for pediatric patients.

Because of its relatively large size and a configuration designed for adults, a posterior cervical plate is probably not appropriate for use in a pediatric patient under the age of 10. A better way to manage an unstable subaxial cervical spine from the posterior direction is to place pedicle or pars screws at the appropriate level and join them with a top-loading rod construct. The rod constructs are sized appropriately for children and are highly versatile. It is the author's opinion that pedicle or pars screws can be routinely placed in the cervical spine in children as young as the age of 4. Further work in this area is necessary to determine appropriate indications and techniques for placing these constructs in children.

## Cable and Wiring Techniques

A rigid anterior plate or posterior rod system may not work in some very young patients requiring cervical fusion because of size or age constraints. In other cases, a posterior bone-and-cable fusion can augment or support an anterior cervical construct (**Fig. 7–7**). In those instances, a posterior bone-and-wire (or bone-and-cable) fusion will provide both internal support and a fusion

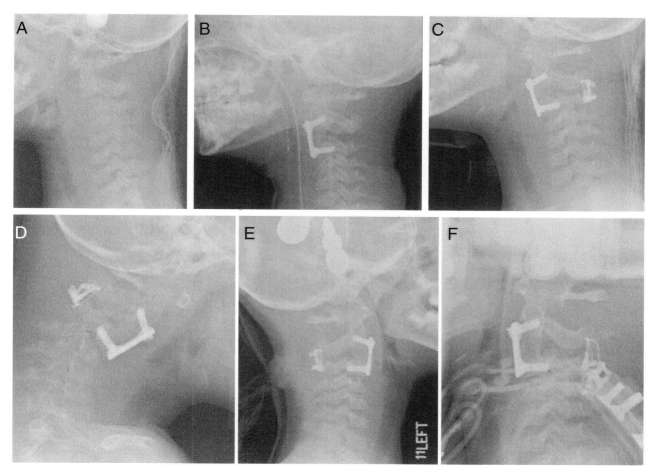

**Figure 7–7**  A 7-year-old girl injured in a motor vehicle accident. **(A)** Plain lateral cervical spine film showing severe C2–C3 distraction and subluxation injury. **(B)** Plain lateral cervical spine film, showing initial anterior cervical diskectomy and fusion construct from the anterior direction, using a Short Stature Anterior Cervical Spine Locking Plate (Synthes, Inc., West Chester, PA). **(C)** Plain lateral cervical spine film, showing addition of posterior bone-and-cable construct and the initial anterior construct. **(D)** Plain lateral cervical spine film taken 6 weeks after surgery, showing severe angulation and subluxation at C3–C4. Note solid bony arthrodesis between C2 and C3 anteriorly. **(E)** Plain lateral cervical spine film, taken with the patient in tong-traction to facilitate realignment. **(F)** Plain lateral cervical spine film, showing the patient in a halo with extension of her posterior fusion from C2 down to C4. She ultimately fused 3 months after surgery.

substrate. These techniques are suitable for either single- or multilevel fusions. Typically, rib graft is harvested for fusion, but posterior iliac crest graft is sometimes used instead. These constructs have the advantage that they may grow with the patient over time. Many different types of posterior cervical wiring techniques have been described over the years,[8] almost all of which were originally meant for adult patients. A few variations of these techniques are useful in children. The author's preferred technique is to use rib, titanium multistranded cable (Songer cable, Medtronic Sofamor Danek), and titanium disks that accept

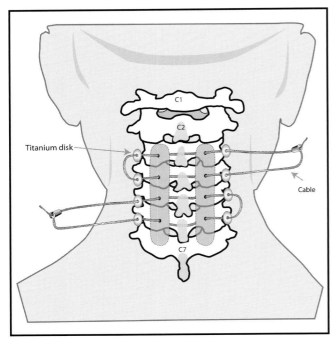

**Figure 7–8**    Multilevel cervical fusion (using rib and cable with titanium disks).

the cable through a screw thread-hole (**Fig. 7–8**). The titanium disks thus protect the rib grafts from being cut by the cable. This construct is strong and versatile and has a very high chance of fusion when augmented with a hard cervical collar or halo orthosis.

## ◆ Bone Graft Materials

The two primary sources of bone graft material for subaxial cervical fusion procedures are autograft and allograft. Autograft may be harvested from several locations, including the anterior iliac crest for anterior procedures and rib or posterior iliac crest for posterior cervical procedures. Autograft is used with a high degree of success in cervical arthrodeses. It is the gold standard in cervical spine surgery. Allograft is available in tricortical iliac crest wedges or femoral struts. For the purposes of pediatric cervical spine surgery, allograft tricortical iliac crest wedges are most appropriate. It has been shown that posterior cervical onlay allograft fusions in children lead to unsuccessful results.[9,10] This technique is not recommended; however, allograft used in an anterior interbody position is highly successful in the pediatric population.[11] To summarize, allograft tricortical iliac wedge at each level is recommended for single- or multilevel anterior cervical diskectomy, whereas autograft anterior iliac crest is recommended for single- or multilevel anterior cervical corpectomy. Rib or posterior iliac crest is the recommended substrate for posterior cervical fusion.

## ◆ External Orthoses

With modern techniques of internal fixation, the vast majority of pediatric patients do not require external immobilization after surgical stabilization of the cervical spine. Occasionally, a patient may require a soft or hard cervical collar for comfort, from which they may be rapidly weaned. The exceptions are patients who are too young or too small to accept internal stabilization or cases when the patient shows gross instability at three or more cervical levels. In those cases, it would be prudent to place the patient in an external halo orthosis postoperatively to supplement whatever internal construct has been placed.

## ◆ Postoperative Follow-up

After an anterior or posterior cervical fusion procedure, careful and timely follow-up is critical. Plain lateral and anteroposterior cervical spine films should be taken on the first postoperative day to determine whether the instrumentation and graft material are in an appropriate location. Monthly plain lateral cervical spine x-rays are taken to follow the fusion process and are discontinued when a solid arthrodesis is documented. This usually occurs 3 to 4 months after surgery, although there is a tendency toward earlier fusions using dynamic cervical plates. Once a successful fusion is demonstrated, yearly films are obtained until the patient stops growing.

## ◆ Advanced Subaxial Cervical Spine Fusion Techniques

Because the author uses standard surgical techniques and approaches for the vast majority of his subaxial cervical fusion procedures, they will not be reviewed here. They include anterior cervical diskectomy and fusion with plating, as well as anterior cervical corpectomy and fusion with plating.

### References

1. McAfee P, Bohlman H, Riley L, et al. The anterior retropharyngeal approach to the upper part of the cervical spine. J Bone Joint Surg Am 1987;69:1371–1383
2. Vardiman A, Dickman C, Sonntag V. Modified anterolateral retropharyngeal approach to the craniovertebral junction. In: Dickman C, Spetzler R, Sonntag V, eds. Surgery of the Craniovertebral Junction. New York: Thieme; 1998:419–431
3. Caspar W, Barbier DD, Klara PM. Anterior cervical fusion and Caspar plate stabilization for cervical trauma. Neurosurgery 1989;25:491–502
4. Epstein N. Anterior cervical dynamic ABC plating with single level corpectomy and fusion in forty-two patients. Spinal Cord 2003;41:153–158
5. Balabhadra R, Kim D, Zhang H. Anterior cervical fusion using dense cancellous allografts and dynamic plating. Neurosurgery 2004;54:1405–1411

6. Roy-Camille R, Saillant G, Mazel C. Internal fixation of the unstable cervical spine by a posterior osteosynthesis with plates and screws. In: Cervical Spine Research Society, ed. The Cervical Spine. Philadelphia: JB Lippincott; 1989:390–403

7. Liu J, Das K. Posterior fusion of the subaxial cervical spine: indications and techniques. Neurosurg Focus 2001;10(4):Article 7, 1–8

8. Abdu WA, Bohlman HH. Techniques of subaxial posterior cervical spine fusions: an overview. Orthopedics 1992;15:287–295

9. Smith MD, Phillips WA, Hensinger RN. Complications of fusion to the upper cervical spine. Spine 1991;16:702–705

10. Smith MD, Phillips WA, Hensinger RN. Fusion of the upper cervical spine in children and adolescents: an analysis of 17 patients. Spine 1991;16:695–701

11. Brockmeyer D, Apfelbaum R, Tippets R, Walker M, Carey L. Pediatric cervical spine instrumentation using screw fixation. Pediatr Neurosurg 1995;22:147–157

# Index

Note: Page numbers followed by f indicate figures.

# *Journal of Neurosurgery*

1224 WEST MAIN STREET, SUITE 450
CHARLOTTESVILLE, VIRGINIA 22903
TELEPHONE: (434) 924-5503 • FAX: (434) 924-2702 • EMAIL: jneuro@virginia.edu
www.thejns-net.org

## *Journal of Neurosurgery*
### Book Review Guidelines

1. Please include the answers to the following two questions with your review.
   a. Is the price appropriate for this book?
   b. Does the title accurately reflect the contents?

2. Please limit the review to no more that 5 pages , double spaced.

3. Please e-mail the review as an attachment to eck9n@virginia.edu.

4. All reviews are due 30 days of receipt of the book.

5. If you have any questions, please feel free to contact Evelyn Kessler at 1-434- 924-2204, email: eck9n@virginia.edu

# Journal of Neurosurgery

1224 WEST MAIN STREET, SUITE 450
CHARLOTTESVILLE, VIRGINIA 22903
TELEPHONE: (434) 924-5503 • FAX: (434) 924-2702 • E-MAIL: jneuro@virginia.edu
www.thejns-net.org

December 5, 2005

Renee Osterdock, M.D.
11234 Anderson St., Rm 2562B
loma Linda CA 92354

Dear Dr. Osterdock, M.D.

Thank you for agreeing to review the enclosed book entitled *Advanced Pediatric Craniocervical Surgery*, by Douglas L. Brockmeyer, (list price $129.95). We recognize the amount of time and effort that will be required on your part to provide us with your review, and we are most appreciative. The book, of course, is yours to keep.

In writing your review, please follow the attached guidelines.

Sincerely Yours,

*Evelyn Kessler*

Evelyn Kessler
Book Review Coordinator

Encl.